from Borderline to *Baseline*

9 KEY STEPS TO MANAGE YOUR BPD AND START LOVING YOUR LIFE

Julie Ann Ford

ISBN: 978-19-5-036748-1

Published by

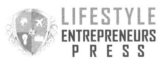

LIFESTYLE
ENTREPRENEURS
P R E S S

If you are interested in publishing through Lifestyle Entrepreneurs Press, write to: *Publishing@LifestyleEntrepreneursPress.com*

Publications or foreign rights acquisition of our catalog books. Learn More: *www.LifestyleEntrepreneursPress.com*

Printed in the USA

This wholehearted dedication goes out to incredible humans without whom this book, not to mention this life, would not have been possible ~ starting with my most amazing dad and mom, whom I adore and love. Brianna Elizabeth, "She Who Pulls Me Through," who has grown into a beautiful and brilliant woman and my beautiful sisters Tammy and Tracey. To those handful of friends who I call my lifers, a.k.a. my life preservers, thank you for always keeping me afloat. To many health care professionals over the years from coast to coast– most especially to both Dr. Ds for saving my life. To those in the fellowship and still trudging, I commend you and thank you for sharing your experience, strength, and hope with me. This book was written to be "someone else's survival guide" and is especially dedicated to those who lost all hope and left us too soon by committing suicide. My friend Rebecca, I miss you so and dedicate this book to you with all of my heart.

Foreword

Julie Ann Ford, the author of this much anticipated, incredibly important book for anyone suffering with borderline personality disorder, is one of the most amazing women I have had the pleasure of knowing. As Ms. Ford's confidant and sometimes counselor, I have been privileged to witness her growth in all aspects of her life – familial, emotional, spiritual and intellectual.

The author has remarkably transformed herself from a woman struggling for many years with overwhelming emotions, physical pain, irrational thoughts, abnormal behavior, and paralyzing anxiety into this exceptionally accomplished, intelligent, controlled and balanced life coach. Albeit Julie has always been brilliant in most endeavours she attempted however, did not seemingly have the confidence to follow through.

As a Trauma and Addiction Counsellor, as well as a close family friend, I have observed up close and personal Julie's miraculous changes over 20 years. Changes that occurred as Julie went to one therapy after another and tried a variety of therapists who used different approaches. She also got involved with various self-help groups. The result of which she has gathered a mix from the different modalities that worked for her. Although difficult, Ms. Fords journey has been incredibly rewarding as she is now able to manage her borderline personality which can be an extremely difficult disorder to live with.

However, in this book Julie has not only described how she manages BPD but has developed a nine-step easy to follow program, FORDitude, that helps with anxiety, fear, irrational thinking, erratic emotions, and behavior. In addition, the program FORDitude comes with a tremendous support, personal coaching, by none other than the author herself, Julie Ford.

If you are someone who is struggling with borderline personality disorder or are still searching for a solution, *Borderline to Baseline* is a must read to assist you in managing your difficult to control symptoms in order to not merely exist but to " make the most of each moment" (p.1).

Borderline to Baseline is invaluable to people living with BPD, their families and the professionals who treat them.

Undoubtedly, *Borderline to Baseline* is an excellent resource for all working in the helping professions.

Marie Helgason, M. Ed.

Contents

Chapter 1

Managing BPD and Your Life Is Possible

"The willingness to accept responsibility for one's own life is the source from which self-respect springs."

Joan Didion

The Real Meaning of BPD

Throughout my battle and recovery from BPD, I had often thought about an alternative acronym for the mental illness, which negatively affected my life for years: But Prefer Death.

I'm sure I wasn't the only one who thought of it. But for me, it often seemed the most accurate explanation for borderline personality disorder and the way it made me feel. This painful truth became even more obvious to me after I came back to consciousness from my last suicide attempt.

I truly didn't think I could deal with the unrelenting pain or continue to search for the will to live anymore, and I swallowed a nearly full ninety-day supply of my sleeping medication. I was in an almost trance-like state when I did so, and afterwards, I felt a strange calm. I desperately wanted the emotional pain, unwarranted shame, self-loathing, and the constant negative and destructive chattering in my head to stop. I had come to refer to this chattering as *the Judge*: it never stopped, and never gave me a moment of peace. *The Judge* presided over me, my every thought, often my impulses, and my regretful decisions.

I felt that if the only way I could stop the pain, noise, and constant confusion was to kill myself, I could justify it. I truly felt, at that time, that in the long run, I would be doing everyone in my life a favour. I thought that it would hurt them initially, but that more pain would result from the embarrassment and shame I caused them in my current state. I told myself they would all be better off without me and the grief I caused them. I didn't want to cause them any further pain from having to deal with my mental health issues and my behaviours.

Back then, I often felt as though I was watching my actions and behaviours from an outsider's perspective, yet I was completely helpless to stop myself. It felt like watching a train speeding down a track, but by the time it realized that the rails had a break, it was too late for the train to stop. You could do nothing but watch helplessly as it continued at full speed and began lifting off the tracks. And when it did, all you could do was squeeze your eyes shut and hope for the best. I absolutely hated feeling that way. Truthfully, I have not enjoyed most of the experiences I have had in my life. For me, there was no middle ground, and my reactions were hair trigger, which made being around me challenging to say the least. That's why I convinced myself that my family would be better off without me and all of the "stuff" I brought with me.

I had seriously attempted suicide several times before, but each time, I was unable to go through with it. My only wish was that I could make it look like an accident because I desperately wanted to protect my daughter and my mother from the truth. But on that day, with that bottle of sleeping pills, there was no turning back. Little did I know, my

Creator had other plans for me and would not allow me to die. So, when I came to two days later, I was not happy about waking at all.

I had fantasized about committing suicide, on nearly a daily basis, as far back as I can remember. I was born feeling wrong and unwanted, and it grew into a true hatred for myself. I hated how I felt most of the time, and not surprisingly, I hated most aspects of my life. I didn't really know who I was, except that I was "too much" for most people, and I was determined to do something to address what was missing in my life.

Since my diagnosis in 2010, I have spent a lot of time in my recovery from borderline personality disorder. During that time, I have come to believe that the reason I am still here is to be able to share my message of recovery through writing this book and developing FORDitude. I want to share my experience, strength, and hope with others who are still struggling – it is my great honour to be able to do so.

Today, I have done my best to adopt a "make the most of each moment" attitude. Time is such a precious commodity and is in such limited supply. Time is the one thing in life that we can't get more of, and I lost so much of it while I was barely existing in this world. What time I didn't waste, I was wishing away.

You may still be struggling and searching for a solution because nothing has worked well enough or helped you manage your BPD so far. You might feel that time is passing you by and that nothing is really helping you feel any better. Maybe you feel that nothing is changing in your mind to allow you to feel like you can manage things in your world for more than a day, or a few at best. That was how it used to be for my client Olivia.

I have come to know Olivia quite well over the past couple of months that we've been working together. She has shared with me that she would get glimpses of how it could be, of how it could feel, and then it would all fall apart again and again. She would find herself back in the same place of hopelessness, and the harsh reality would set in that this was likely how it would always be for her. *Or so she thought.*

Glimpses of Life Living with BPD: Olivia's Story

Having BPD was hell on earth, in my experience, and I knew as soon as I first began talking to and working with Olivia that it had been her experience also – only she was still living there daily. She told me of how she never felt like she fit in anywhere, especially with her family. She remembered feeling incredible love and affection towards people; however, she couldn't trust that it would be returned – at least not without many strings and conditions attached. This was always unspoken – yet she assumed and felt that she somehow knew it to be true. Later, she would be proven right time and again when her needs would be overlooked in favor of her parents meeting their own first – whether it be an extra case of beer taking the place of a meal not eaten, or another night spent in her cold, dark, and scary house alone while her parents were out having fun at one place or another. Who knew where the wind may have carried them off to that night or what time they may eventually end up back home.

Olivia shared that she lived in a constant state of over-whelming confusion, uncertainty, and fear that she was unlovable, unworthy of love, and that the only thing she was consistently capable of was letting people down. She felt she did that very well. Olivia told me how her mother was especially critical of her, and very demanding of her from schoolwork to chores around the house. She seemed to constantly disappoint her parents by not doing what they wanted, her ex-boyfriend was quick to point out all her shortcomings, and even her friends said how she could be so hot and cold. It was easier sometimes to keep to herself and not look to anyone for anything, especially understanding of any kind.

Dysfunctional Childhood

Both of Olivia's parents were alcoholics, which makes for a very challenging environment for a kid to live in, especially when you are a child with an undiagnosed personality dis-order. Growing up in an alcoholic home is kind of like being in a school playground that is made of jelly and trying to stand up straight. Just when you think you have it mastered, you realize that you must get off the ground fast and jump up on the jungle gym. But there's always someone sitting at the top waiting. You never quite know who you'll meet at the top of the jungle gym, or what that person's reaction will be on that day, but they always look like your parents, even though that person could act like your best friend or your worse foe. You never know until you are up there, and there is nothing you can do except hope it will over quickly – whatever *it* was. You may have met with sober, remorseful parents who didn't mind you being around so much. You may have met with drunk parents, whose only concern was getting more liquor and did not ensure their child being fed or taken care of.

Olivia and I have talked about those early, confusing, and frightening experiences, and what it was like not to be able to rely on either of her parents for comfort or support. It is an incredibly tough environment to grow up in, especially for an anxious child. It caused Olivia great confusion, uncertainty, and instability, and created irrational fears and loneliness within her. This was especially true for Olivia as she was the only child in her family and had no one else to spend time with at home while she was growing up. She had tried to talk to both of her parents many times over the years, and it didn't improve anything. This lack of connection and healthy bond with her parents denied her the ability to learn coping skills from her family of origin. She did not learn how to be a good mom for her daughter, Rosie, as she did not have positive role models herself. She discovered this while we were working together, and it has allowed her to be much more compassionate and understanding with herself when she gets impatient and frustrated with Rosie. She can now see how her past negatively affects her relationship with Rosie. Now that Olivia has had an opportunity to process and understand the missing role models and examples from her life, she has been noticing a big improvement in her parenting relationship with Rosie.

Olivia's Traumas

Olivia revealed to me that she had been raped by a nineteen-year-old family friend when she was thirteen. He took her virginity, and Olivia did not tell anyone about her sexual assaults. It happened the first time she tried smoking weed, and he forced himself on her while she laid on the kitchen floor in tears. She was unable to stop his assault no matter how many times she asked him. She is still traumatized and devastated by the event and the fact that her virginity was robbed from her.

She told me of another time, when she was fourteen, that she was passed out drunk and woke up in the bathroom of her aunt's house with her much older male cousin's fingers inside of her. To this day, she is still so deeply affected by this that she has to tell her boyfriends to *never* touch her or her "privates" intimately in her sleep because to say it won't be well received would be an understatement. Her entire sexual being has been hugely and negatively influenced by these awful experiences. She mistakenly carried a lot of guilt and shame for years until she was able to reframe what happened to her, and finally place the blame properly on the shoulders of the perpetrators – where it had belonged the whole time.

Suicide Attempts

Before she gave birth to her daughter, Rosie, she had made two serious attempts at suicide and, thankfully, was unsuccessful. She told me that it was not a cry for attention, she simply could not tolerate the pain and constant emotional chaos and turmoil in her head, and she just did not want to live anymore.

Since the birth of her daughter, she has a new lease on life, and she has committed to living her life fully, and under any and all conditions and circumstances.

Rosie – Her daughter and Heart

Rosie is Olivia's four-year-old daughter, the apple of her eye, and the reason for her continuing to "fight the good fight," as she puts it. Olivia and Rosie's dad, Rick, a semi-successful musician, are separated, and Rosie happily spends most of her time with her mom. She is a sweet and precocious little girl who I have had the pleasure of meeting several times. She has a smile that could melt your heart. Olivia really wants to be the best mother she can be for Rosie and is willing to put in the work and make some big changes in her lifestyle and thinking to facilitate making the most of my program and her life. I am so pleased to see her putting the program into daily practice and seeing the changes starting to take place – for both her and Rosie.

The Path to FORDitude

I was first introduced to Olivia through our mutual friend, Lisa, who asked if I would be willing to talk to Olivia. The three of us got together, and I shared with Olivia that I was writing a book and finalizing the creation of a program, which I was using successfully to manage BPD in my own life. I had decided at that point that I wanted to call the program FORDitude.

What started out as a coffee turned into well over an hour of talking and Olivia's very keen interest in beginning to work with me so she could learn what I have spent the better part of the past ten years dedicating my life to searching out. What I found was being able to learn all that I could about BPD and a commitment to the conscious action of managing my mind and building my connection to Source or Creator. I will share, here and now, some of what I shared with Olivia that day.

I learned that everything I put into my mind and body affects me in ways I didn't know were possible and with such far reaching implications. I could not have known what they were until I eliminated them and no longer felt their poisonous and toxic effects. I learned that I am not what I think, despite what I thought – if that makes sense! And yes, it does so matter what you think, say, and do. Giving of yourself to be of service to others is an important part of your job here, and it's the little things that you do that will add up to become the big differences because there is *no* magic pill to take (I am not referring to necessary medications, of course), and there are no short cuts to anyplace worth going to. At the start, the middle, and the end of every day, there is you, and no matter where you go, there you are. So, it's time to get good with you because you are what you have to work with. You are loved, you are enough, and you are in the right place, right now. And I am right here with you.

Good Prognosis Diagnosis

On, now, to some fantastic news and just a of hint of the good things you will find out as you continue reading this book. Contrary to a lot of misinformation out there concerning this often-perplexing disorder, let me reassure you that having borderline personality disorder is the good prognosis diagnosis. What do I mean? Below, I have listed the nine symptoms of BPD:

1. **Fear of abandonment:** Those of us with BPD are often plagued with thoughts, real and imagined, of being abandoned or left alone. This can result in unwarranted fears and efforts to keep someone close, but instead our erratic and confusing behaviours will often drive them away. It is also not uncommon for us to preemptively end relationships, even if it was not the intention of the other person to end the relationship in the first place. It is a maladaptive protective mechanism used that ultimately hurts us.

2. **Unstable relationships:** Those of us with BPD are prone to having tumultuous relationships and lacking a middle ground where we swing from idealization to devaluation, anger, and hate.

3. **Unclear or shifting self-image:** Our sense of self is unstable and as such we can hate ourselves. With no real idea of who we are or what we like or want, we often change looks, jobs, lovers, and even religions.

4. **Impulsive, self-destructive behaviors:** You may engage in dangerous, pleasure seeking behaviors when upset, which could look like substance abuse of drugs or alcohol, overspending, reckless driving, casual and risky sex, compulsive eating, or any other behavior that helps you to temporarily feel better but has negative consequences in the long-term.

5. **Self-harm**: Self harming behaviors such as cutting and/ or suicidal thoughts and behavior are very common for those of us with BPD.

6. **Extreme emotional swings**: Extreme mood swings are common for those of us with BPD. You can feel happy one moment only to become despondent the next, and it will take you much longer to return to feeling okay. The little things that others easily brush off can send you into an emotional tailspin, lasting from minutes to hours.

7. **Chronic feelings of emptiness**: You may have feelings of "nothingness", being nobody, and having a big hole in you, or a void, that can't be filled. Many of us have tried unsuccessfully with food, sex, alcohol and drugs, but to no avail – nothing ever feels truly satisfying.

8. **Explosive anger**: For those of us with BPD, struggling with anger and a bad temper is a big concern. You may have trouble controlling your actions once the top is off the pot, so to speak, and can become consumed with rage. You may also be like how I was and turn that anger inwards for fear of what could happen if that rage is unleashed – it's like a ticking time bomb inside of you.

9. **Feeling out of touch with reality or suspicious**: You may, under extreme stress, experience episodes of feeling foggy or spaced out as if you're outside of your own body. This is known as disassociation. You may also experience paranoia, suspicion, and question others' motives.

To be diagnosed as Borderline, you must exhibit five of these nine symptoms. The cessation (stopping) of these symptoms/behaviors that identify BPD means that you are no longer considered to have the mental illness/disorder. With consistency and regular practice of new, positive, healthy replacement behaviours, you can, and will, learn how to live your life in a way that is not characterized by the symptoms of BPD. You can have the same freedom and happiness I have experienced and enjoy.

Olivia's Continued Progress

Today, so long as Olivia does the work each day that *she* has decided is important for her to manage her mind and her life, she can and will be able to accomplish anything she puts her heart into. If, however, nothing was to change, nothing *will* change, and the chances of her finishing her degree will be slim, working as anything but a server will be unlikely, and dealing with chronic pain for the rest of her life will also be likely. I know that Olivia is hungry for a change and is willing to take a chance to be happy and to do the work to make the rest of her life the best of her life – are you?

Bottom Line

Based on the research and information available to mental health professionals today, most believe that the cause of borderline personality disorder is a combination of inherited or internal biological factors and external environmental factors, such as adverse childhood experiences (ACEs). I will talk much more about this, the meaning behind ACE scores, and the impact it has had on my life in Chapter 6.

As children, we do not choose the nature of our upbringing, but it has had a huge impact on our lives today. The information available to us today, from current research, shows that adverse childhood events are linked directly to future health conditions. It is my hope that this explanation will allow for more people to begin looking at their mental health and addiction issues and realize that it is not a matter of willpower or choice as has been erroneously thought for a long time. I pray that the correct knowledge brought forward to the public's view will reframe the old thinking and negative stigma that has been associated with mental health and addiction. I hope the climate will be more open and receptive to encourage people to be proud to be in recovery – to step out of the darkness and stand in their light with support and hope for the future.

You are not responsible for a lot of the things that have happened in your life or for the fact that you have BPD; however, I do believe that you are responsible for what you do about it now. You *are* a worthy human being capable of loving, caring, healing, sharing, learning, and choosing to do differently than you've done in the past – *and* you can start right now. I am asking you to take the time to read through this book and see if the FORDitude Daily Action Program resonates with you, as I believe it will. It is not an instant fix – there is no such thing, but it is the culmination of small things that over time will make a big difference in your life when you believe that you are worth it. And in case no one has told you lately, you are worth it! You can and will learn how to *finally* manage your mind, BPD, and life using the FORDitude Daily Action Program.

Chapter 2

My Battle with BPD and Declaring Myself Victorious

"I count him braver who overcomes his desires than him who conquers his enemies; for the hardest victory is over self".

Aristotle

"Keep coming back, it works *if* you work it – and *you are worth it!*"

So, I guess it's all true what they say, or, more to the point, what I say at the end of the recovery meetings I attend. While holding hands in a circle, after we close with the serenity prayer, it just automatically comes out of my mouth, and, eventually, it made its way into my subconscious, until I one day I started believing it.

I will give most of the credit to Donald, a recovery friend of mine who has sadly passed away. He had a tough life from day one and struggled for years with medical issues. He even ended up in a wheelchair, but he never lost his positive spirit. And despite his life of adversity and dealing with more hardships than I could imagine, he had years of sobriety. He taught me how to live with dignity and grace, no matter what life throws at you. At our recovery meetings, after his final stroke, the only thing he said was "Keep coming back. It works if you work it, and you're worth it." After all those years of saying the same thing over and over again, it really does begin to change the old mental tapes and will slowly make new pathways in your brain – especially the brain of this once confused and lost woman. This woman who, growing up, didn't believe that she was worth much of anything at all. How could I be when I knew from my beginning that I was born "wrong"? Well the wrong sex at least. I was not the son Dad really, really wanted.

Born with An Identity Complex

Let me go way back and tell you that I believe that I was born with an identity crisis or complex. I'm not sure what you would have called it, but I just knew how it felt, and it felt horrible. I will introduce myself. I am Julie, and I'm a Grateful Recovering Emotional Alcoholic Today, so I get to say that I'm GREAT under any and all circumstances, whether I feel like a million bucks or a bucket of crap. I've always known that one of the many gifts I was born with is that of being an exceptional communicator. I've just never known how to use it effectively. It, and me, was always too much. I spent my life overcompensating in countless ways to feel like I fit in and belong because I never felt as though I did.

I now understand much more the reasons why I felt like that from birth, and I understand the science behind it, right back to discovering that while I was still in my Mother's womb, her stress, worries, and downright fear about whether or not I would be born a girl or a boy must have weighed heavily on her. So much so, that I believe it is the reason why my birth was delayed. I was due February 2, 1971, and I didn't arrive until March 2, 1971.

But, in typical Julie style, when I did arrive, there was no stopping me. From Mom's first labour pain, I arrived in the world twenty minutes later with the doctor having to run down the hall to make it in time for my delivery. My dad, a handsome Air Force officer pilot with a daredevil attitude and larger than life persona, wanted a son more than anything. Unfortunately for him, I was to be the third of the already agreed upon three children that he and my beautiful Mom were going to have: my two older siblings were both girls. So, when he arrived from Rhode Island, where our family was posted at that time, in a cast and crutches (he had been participating in survival training exercises the previous day and somehow had broken his leg while jumping out of an airplane) to surprise my mom in her hospital room, I don't know who was more surprised – and I'm not really sure "surprised" is the best word to use. I would take on the identity of having been born wrong and as a disappointment, and those are probably the two nicest words I can use to describe my earliest feelings of self.

First Memory

My first memory is from the day that we moved from Rhode Island back to Canada when my father got posted to Ottawa, Ontario. That would've been in the summer of 1973, when I would have just turned two years old. Back then, I know practices were much different concerning children being out and about, so I guess it didn't seem unusual for my parents to allow my older sister, Tammy, who would have been seven at the time, to take care of me and my other sister, Tracey, who was five. We were at a playground at the very top of Dennison Crescent, where we had just moved. I'm not sure how long we were there, as my memories are sketchy from that day, but I do remember the feeling of missing my mom and really wanting to go home to be with her, so I left the playground. I was walking down what turned out to be the wrong side of the Crescent. All of the bungalows were the same – all red brick – and I wasn't able to find which of the houses was ours. I couldn't see the moving truck parked in the driveway.

Lost and Terrified

I don't remember all of the specific details, but I do vividly remember, forty-six years later, how scared I was and the feeling of desperation of not knowing how to get home or if I would ever find my mother. I remember the feelings of being lost and so fearful, sitting on a curb bawling my eyes out.

I don't know how long I sat there, crying, before my father drove up, frantically, and found me. When he did, he didn't react happily; he didn't react nicely at all. I understand why now, as an adult. I can understand that the fear he felt at not knowing where I was, being frightened for my safety, and unsure about my whereabouts caused him to respond with anger. Unfortunately, I was the recipient of that behaviour, and his actions when he saw me were not to console his terrified two-year-old and embrace her with reassurance and love. Instead, he yelled at me, shook me hard, and chastised me for walking away from my sisters at the playground and scaring my mother half to death. He never once thought for a moment that his thoughtless words and actions would be a pivotal and defining moment in my life. They would, in fact, set the stage for my battle with identity disturbance and my complete disconnection from myself and my ability to like myself or know who I was. Forget the notion or concept of loving myself – that was such a foreign concept unimaginable to me.

Truth be known, I spent most of my life fearing myself and who I really was. I didn't know who or what I was until I learned about why the traumas and other awful things happened to me. I felt that I must be a bad person deep inside, otherwise why would such awful things have happened to me – more than once? When a child has no one safe and reliable to talk to and confide in, that child creates stories about herself to help try and make sense of what is happening in her life and why it is happening, and, sadly, there are no happy endings.

I can remember thinking that if there was a "God" he must not have liked me, and I must have been a really bad person deep inside, otherwise, my Dad would not act the way he did with me. I even knew that it was different with me than it was with my two sisters. He was not the same with them as he was with me. And he got really, really upset with me when he drank. He never hit me, but his words could cut deeper than any knife. I remember feeling so confused about why he didn't seem to want me around, and I was always trying to get his approval and attention. I only ever succeeded in getting his negative attention and that never ended well for me. I spent a lot of my childhood hiding, sometimes in the house sometimes in the outbuildings or in the woods that bordered our property, but a lot of the time I hid in plain sight. I always felt that even though I would be in the same room as my family, watching TV or having dinner, no one ever really listened to me or understood me, and I certainly didn't feel like I fit in.

My Trauma

Some of us have tragically been the victim of others' unwarranted and unconscionable behaviours. I myself have been sexually assaulted several times and carried the shame and guilt with me for years, not realizing it was *not* my fault. I didn't tell anyone about it – and really, who could I have talked to about it when these things happened to me beginning at the age of ten? Not my parents, sadly. During those years, they weren't available to me, as they were dealing with their own issues, and I didn't have anywhere else to turn. Only in the last decade would I learn that, at worst, I was only guilty of making a bad decision. That was to drink or do drugs, but *never* did I do anything to deserve what was done to me. I now understand the consequences of having BPD and that it meant I had nonexistent self-esteem and huge abandonment issues. I would unknowingly gravitate to risky people and situations in an attempt to try and find love and acceptance anywhere and from anyone.

This knowledge has helped me to heal to a large degree, and put things in perspective, but I will forever be scarred by what those sick men did to me, and their actions will affect me negatively for the rest of my life. The more work I have done over the years, the less their behaviour and actions affect me today.

Hurtful Things Taken to Heart

"You're too much."

"You're so intense."

"You go from zero to sixty in one second."

"Stop being so sensitive."

"You're a troublemaker."

"We have to walk on our tippy toes around you."

"You are too emotional."

I consistently replay these quotes in my head. The people who spoke them have come in and out of my life – my family members are some of them. I feel my emotions and feelings far more deeply and for far longer than most people; although, on the surface that may not sound entirely life altering, it's crippling. Marsha Linehan, PhD and the founder and developer of dialectical behavioral therapy, likens borderlines to having third degree emotional burns because we feel everything so intensely. When a friend or someone shares something impactful with me, very often, my body will instantly respond in goosebumps covering me entirely from head to toe! And trust me, there is no worse feeling than knowing that you are the odd ball in any and every group. I was always the one who couldn't control her reactions to what was happening. I would react instantaneously, and 99 percent of the time, I would regret my reactions. To say they weren't thought out would be an understatement.

My out of control emotions would take centre stage, and inevitably take everyone hostage. I was often told that it seemed like I was trying to get everyone's attention when, in fact, that was the exact opposite of what I truly wanted.

I really wanted to hide and not be seen, but at that point, I had zero ability to control my tears and my rage. People would comment all the time that I was so sensitive, like I didn't already know, seemingly expecting that the knowledge would help me toughen up, but it only served to further hurt and invalidate me and how I was feeling. I was incapable of explaining to anyone that it wasn't my choice to feel or express myself the way I did – quite the contrary. If I had my choice, I would certainly *not* be choosing to conduct myself this way at all. Years ago, it was even more difficult because we didn't have the resources that are available now online to share with family and friends to help educate them about what BPD is and what it is like for us to live with the disorder.

Medical Misfit

From a very early age, I took on the role of the medical misfit and was chronically unwell a lot. If there was anyone in our family or my group of friends who was sick or got injured, it was me. I was the consummate tomboy, no surprise there, with absolutely no fear of trying something new, and I would do anything on a dare. So, you can imagine that led to some pretty nasty scrapes and bangs. In all seriousness, it is a wonder I didn't end up hospitalized with more than just a cast or in for a scheduled operation. I had the standard and expected brushes with childhood illnesses, and then graduated to a broken wrist. I was goofing around, and ended up with getting my foot crushed in a conveyor belt. I contracted plantar warts from the swimming pool – most people get one or two, I had to undergo surgery on both feet to have all 22 warts dealt with, 10 on one foot, and 12 on the other. I went on to have two surgeries on my right knee, which was my jumping knee from when I was figure skating, three abdominal surgeries for endometriosis (the first of which at the age of sixteen, ultimately resulting in a hysterectomy at the age of twenty-seven), a breast reduction, a skull tumor removed, and in an effort to deal with chronic sinusitis, the sinus surgery I had and went horribly wrong when the cleaning instrument slipped and cracked the membrane and caused cerebral fluid to seep into my sinus cavity, resulting in months of inactivity to ensure the grafting healed properly. The real troublemakers and constants were always the bad headaches and upset stomach aches that accompanied me most of my life.

I wasn't supposed to be able to get pregnant and have children at all due to the extreme endometriosis that I was diagnosed with at 14 years of age. It is one of the leading causes of infertility, so becoming pregnant with my baby naturally really was miraculous – however – I could easily write another book about the ensuing pregnancy, morning sickness, induction, delivery, episiotomy, sugar water, nipple confusion, breast feeding challenges, high needs baby sleeping only 20 minutes, and ultimately, painful intercourse leading me back into to Operating Room for reconstructive surgery six months after birth, then post-surgical infection and readmission for five days for IV antibiotic drip. Pleasant experience doesn't exactly describe it.

Then came the fateful day in February 1997. I was walking into work at the bank, and as is typical on the east coast of Canada, the parking lot was white. Not with snow, but with the residue from the salt that is spread generously in parking lots as it gets very slippery with both ice and snow that time of year. I couldn't see the difference in height as I made my way across the parking lot, and my toe caught on a spot with about a two-inch height difference. I lost my balance and fell forward. Trying not to fall on my face, I ended up turning and landed on my right shoulder, which completely knocked the wind out of me. I couldn't get up and certainly had no inkling then as to what had just happened or the impact that it would have on my life.

One of my colleagues had been outside the door. He saw me fall and came over to help me up. I managed to compose myself, catch my breath, literally brush myself off, and went in to work my shift that day. Other than ruining my leather jacket and shaking me up, I didn't think I was any worse for wear. Thankfully, someone had the foresight to suggest that an incident report be written up because my fall had happened at the workplace.

I started to get a headache that evening and was quite sore and a little stiff by the time I went to bed that night. I awoke at about three o'clock in the morning with agonizing pain and was experiencing my first of what would be many muscle spasms in my neck and upper back. I had never experienced pain like that before, and I was hysterical. I didn't know what to do. This was the beginning of the end of my life as I had known it, and to say I wasn't prepared for what was to come would be a major understatement.

I had just bought a house, and my daughter Brianna, the light of my life, my blessing, had just turned four a couple of weeks before. I went from being a very active hands-on mom, to one who could no longer even pick her up. Forget getting down on the ground and rolling around playing like we had done so often before. I would suffer from debilitating headaches that would force me to shut myself in my darkened room for hours, if not longer at times, and worst of all, I was away from my daughter. It would only be years later that I would fully realize the devasting impact that my injury had on Brianna and how she still suffers from anxious and irrational fears based on thoughts that she was going to lose me.

Thankfully, because I had a great job with a good employer, I had benefits and went on short-term and long-term disability. Within six months, I was prescribed antidepressant medication to cope with all of the negativity, uncertainty, and detrimental changes that took place in all aspects of my life and career. I dealt with all the financial, mental, and physical changes, not to mention, the pain, fear, loss, and grieving of the life I had. I was angry because I had worked so hard for everything I had built for Brianna and me, and I felt helpless and hopeless. I wasn't accepting it well – not at all.

Eighteen months later, I was not responding to treatment and not getting any better, so I was seen by a specialist and diagnosed with fibromyalgia. It would be another fifteen years before I would find out that I was not properly treated after my accident. Only one of the two whiplash injuries that I sustained that day was treated. I had suffered both forward and sideways flexation whiplash injuries from my head being flung forward initially and then when I turned sideways to land on my side. My head also had a sideways flexation, which for the next several years would be the cause of more pain and suffering on a level that was magnified and amplified due to the meninges and scar tissue at the brain stem. It caused massive issues resulting in brain fog, chronic fatigue, severe emotionality (as if my BPD wasn't enough already) and a plethora of other related symptoms that added to the struggles, making it virtually impossible for me to work. God knows I tried, though. I was asked to go back on disability by my managers, but I did not want to be home on disability. That was not what I wanted for me or my life – *not* at all.

I made many trips to the hospital over the years, often brought on by a migraine or a massive muscle spasm, for intravenous muscle relaxants and pain management. It was not my idea of a good time, trust me. One time comes to mind when I was taking Bri to visit her Dad in Prince Edward Island, where he lived on his large potato farm, and I went to my pal Victoria's house after I had dropped Bri off. I wanted to call Bri, as I normally did, and make sure that she was settled in okay. As I reached across my front to get my cell phone out of my purse, all of muscles in my back and surrounding my rib cage went into spasm. I couldn't breathe, and I dropped like a rock to the floor. Victoria called 9-1-1, and I was taken by an ambulance to the hospital for treatment. I was released later that day. What was supposed to be a fun, relaxing weekend break for me, was not so much. Through that experience, I learned that I am prone to carrying a lot of tension in my body. It was a perfect storm for becoming a prime candidate for muscle spasms. It is so true that knowledge is power.

BPD Diagnosis

It was only when I was given a completed copy of my dis-ability application form from my physician, Dr. Dixon, that I learned of my Border Personality Disorder diagnosis. I was 39 years old and had spent the vast majority of my life suffering from mental illness, yet knowing I wasn't fully "crazy", but not knowing what exactly was wrong with me. I had such an unexplainable range of feelings and emotions when I saw "Borderline Personality Disorder" in writing. It was the answer to so many questions from so many years. Now I finally knew what was wrong in my head and why I felt the way I have all of my life – can you say hallelujah! I felt such relief wash over for me and for a few minutes it was a relief to know what was going on – there was a name for what I had, and now I could get started dealing with the diagnosis, right? Then, the reality set in, and I realized a couple of things in that moment.

Why hadn't she told me before that I had BPD?

Since I could remember, I had experienced suicidal thoughts and behaviors, impulsive behaviour, intense and dysfunctional relationships, feelings of persistent emptiness or boredom, a major identity crisis, and a damaged view of self. This affected my emotions, values, moods, and relation-ships, and caused me to have addictive issues and substance abuse and anger issues that resulted in extreme guilt and remorse, extreme depression, anxiety, or irritability. These feelings could persist for hours or days. Sometimes I would be left feeling dissociated, watching myself like an observer.

What did having BPD mean for me? I didn't know enough about it to understand, but what I did feel was still the sense of relief of finally knowing. But then I got fearful and retreated into depression and isolation again. I didn't say anything or tell anyone about my diagnosis for several months after finding out myself. Before I was comfortable talking about it, I did a lot of research and began to learn as much as I could to understand it and when I did, somehow for me, that knowing became freedom.

Since my diagnosis, I have come to understand that a large number of doctors do not provide a diagnosis of borderline personality disorder to their patients. I do not agree with this approach as I believe that every person has the right to all information concerning their medical situation, status, and care. It is that individual's right to have access to that knowledge and the ability to gain understanding and awareness of what the disorder is and how it can be treated. If not just for the simple fact that it provided me comfort and reassurance that there is an answer for what I have been experiencing in your life, it can also give me the ability to relate to the symptoms and have peace of mind.

An educational presentation from the National Education Alliance for BPD on stigma surrounding BPD states that on average, one out of forty people who are known to have BPD have not been told by their doctors or clinicians. I believe that everyone has the right to all the information to allow them the opportunity to pursue all options for treatments.

I lived every day with every emotion on the surface, ready to be set off with the slightest provocation, no matter what the circumstances were. When I was happy, I felt euphoric, and when I was angry, I was a monster whose anger I was afraid to let out. I didn't allow myself to get angry because

I couldn't trust myself, and as a result, I ended up getting very sick, mentally, physically and spiritually. I had nothing inside me but a big empty hole in my soul. I had no way of knowing at the time, but because I stuffed down so much anger and unresolved issues, I created a very toxic environment in my body. I lacked any healthy coping skills that would have allowed me to process the areas of outstanding issues, including the festering anger. Unknowingly, I had become a pressure cooker. I developed a range of issues from irritable bowel syndrome, chronic headaches, stomach aches, acid reflux, chronic sinusitis, and the list goes on.

When I was sad, I would get so depressed that I could go "down" for days at a time and literally couldn't talk to anyone – at all. My body and feelings would sometimes simply shut off, and I would become completely disconnected. It would feel as though I had absolutely nothing inside of me – I could not care, I could not feel sad, or any other emotions, and I had no idea how long it would last, when it would happen, or why it would happen only that it would – and it would no longer be my choice. I realize now this is disassociation.

The other part of it was splitting. I was an all or nothing, black or white, go big or stay home kind of girl. I would proudly boast "if you want to run with the big dogs, you can't pee like a puppy." So, if I wasn't going out in a big way, I wasn't even going to bother getting ready.

Putting my disorder into words is impossible, but I will try my best. My mind is a maze and it made me sick to even think of it sometimes. All I would want is to be close to people. I would be desirous of a relationship where I could share love and be safe, but I would become too intense and too much for anybody to handle. So, I'm on my own today, by choice, after finally breaking free of a very unhealthy, codependent marriage.

I suffered every day. I felt overwhelmed all the time. I found it difficult to communicate. What I feel in my heart and in my head doesn't translate. I can love you with my mind, body, and soul while my words are the exact opposite. I would often find that I would simply shut off or shut down and feel absolutely nothing. I always knew that I lacked the ability to feel empathy for anyone who was sick or not feeling well, and I would blame it on the fact that I myself dealt with so much chronic pain on a daily basis that it left little room for me to have compassion and understanding for anyone else. When it came to being a parent, I would be empathetic to my daughter because I was intelligent enough to be able to model the behaviours I witnessed my own mother acting out. I could fake it, and no one was the wiser – except me. And that was always the problem. I always knew how I didn't feel. I just didn't know why I didn't feel those things.

Contrary to what people likely think, it was never about wanting to start drama or seek attention. When I overreact, it is not easy for me to recover, and it takes much longer for me to return to baseline. I hurt, I hurt others, and I am depleted of all energy at the end of the day. I have had to wear masks and create facades to get through, and when I get home, I have nothing left for my family. I was constantly afraid of the idea of being alone – abandonment is hell. I latch onto people and would often let go of them before they could let go of me. Many people believe that I was a mean, nasty, manipulator. My moods changed all the time, so quickly it was hard to keep up with me, and I had zero control over my emotions. I feel everything so deeply, and I have heard it said it's like being born with one less layer of skin, so you not only feel your emotions that much more intensely, but you take in and feel everyone else's emotions around you also so the load is always so heavy to carry.

Things that have Made a Difference in My Healing Journey

There have been countless days and nights I didn't want to be alive, and, with my family history of substance abuse and mental illness, there have been periods of insanity. I was a mess. After sustaining my whiplash injury and dealing with the chronic pain and depression, my fibromyalgia diagnosis, and life, I was abusing alcohol to try and cope with all of my issues. I was on a fast track to nowhere worth going.

Thankfully, when I moved in 2005 from Nova Scotia to British Columbia, I was surrounded by a lot of amazing people in recovery. This is because my dad has been in the fellowship of Alcoholics Anonymous since 1986 and has continued on with his program since he and mom retired to Comox Valley in the early 90s. I met a number of young women who had attained significant sobriety, and I was both intrigued by and impressed with them. Long before I found my own sobriety, I began spending time with a few of these women and came to the realization that I wanted what they had, and I knew that I would need to start changing my old habits.

On my journey of recovery, I constantly faced misunderstanding, judgement, and lack of sympathy concerning my mental illness. It was at times offending, isolating, and discouraging, and it made it difficult to find support. After seeking help, trying medications, and dealing with years of struggle, I eventually found a sense of stability through books. I would choose the book, learn new information, and ultimately find new and better ways to approach my day-to-day life.

Melody Beattie's *Codependent No More*

Codependent No More changed *everything* I understood and knew about relationships, and because of it and her companion daily meditation book, *The Language of Letting Go*, my life changed. I could start each day off on the right foot and set my intention and direction. It always amazes me that I can read the same passage again and learn something new.

Byron Katie's *Loving What Is*

Loving What Is changed how I process what I think and what I used to resist day-to-day, by not accepting things in life as they are. I really found her work to be so meaningful and insightful, and by doing the work, it had a tremendous impact on me and my life. I am forever changed for the better. Many thanks and gratitude to her for helping me learn how to embrace loving what is.

Louise Hay's *You Can Heal Your Life*

You Can Heal Your Life was hugely instrumental in teaching me that I can and will heal my life if I am willing to put the effort and energy that is required into healthy practices of self-care and self-love. I did not have a positive connection with myself to know who I was – forget liking myself – so loving myself was a far-off concept to me. Through affirmations, mirror work, and learning to be gentle and compassionate with myself, I was able to begin the process of accepting myself, which eventually led to me liking myself. Today I am thrilled to say that I love myself, and I did not believe that was ever going to be a reality for me.

Belleruth Naparstek's *Invisible Heroes*

Invisible Heroes: Survivors of Trauma and How They Heal taught me so many important things concerning traumatic events and how to begin recovering from them. I was able to understand my part and, as importantly, what parts weren't mine, including the shame, blame, and such. The imagery and visualization techniques in this book are plentiful and are well worth the cost for the benefit of them alone.

Joseph Murphy's *The Power of the Subconscious Mind*

The Power of the Subconscious Mind was a pivotal learning tool for me to start to understand the scope and power of the subconscious mind. Up until I began reading this incredibly powerful book, I was truly unaware of the full capabilities of the subconscious mind and how underutilized it is in most of us and in our society in general. The book was written in 1963 and, for over fifty years now, it has been one of the bestselling spiritual self-help books, ever. After years of research, he teaches us that a great power is within all of us, and by focusing and redirecting that energy, you can change your destiny. He shares specific practical techniques and prayers that you can use to practice and accomplish these attainable goals.

Andrew Weil, MD's *Natural Health, Natural Medicine*
Natural Health, Natural Medicine is a book that found its way into my possession when I decided to enroll in a correspondence course for a wellness course. I have found that it contains an amazing amount of very practical information for everyday health concerns, and much of what I am sharing with you, I have learned from Dr. Weil and have incorporated into my FORDitude plan.

What I Continue to Do about It

I maintain my daily routine of essential to-dos, which I have developed and put together by integrating key aspects and elements of recovery that I have been involved in over the past decade: psychotherapy, Alcoholics Anonymous (AA), dialectic behavioural therapy (DBT), mindfulness, meditation, etc. This simple, but not to be confused as easy, daily program of action has made the difference in helping me change my old, ineffective habits and patterns of thinking and doing. This has allowed me to forge new pathways in my brain, and I have been able to enjoy a new way forward. I am now living a life worth waking up to every morning, and I am excited about. I can be present for my family, my daughter, my parents, friends, and, most importantly, I can be there today for me – the me I am proud of who I finally know and love. I am willing to put in the work every day because the rewards are so worth the effort required, and I know if I don't do my part, the results will not be there.

Personality Under Development

I took my first Myers Briggs Personality Test about twenty years ago while employed at the Canadian Imperial Bank Commerce Electronic Banking Centre in Halifax, Nova Scotia. I was, to a T, an "Executive" type: Extroverted, Sensing, Thinking, Judging, (ESTJ). A number of months ago, I did the test again, expecting a slightly different result but was shocked to see the extent of the changes that had taken place over the past ten years of excavating through the "stuff that was never mine to begin with". I uncovered that I am truly an "Advocate" Personality type: Introverted, Intuitive, Feeling, Judging (INFJ). People with my personality type tend to see helping others as their purpose in life. Advocates can often be found engaging in rescue efforts and doing charity work. However, their real passion is to get to the heart of the issue so that people need not be rescued at all. Advocates indeed share a unique combination of traits. Advocates find it easy to make connections with others. They have a talent for warm, sensitive language, speaking in human terms, rather than pure logic and facts. These types tend to believe that nothing would help the world so much as using love and compassion to soften the hearts of tyrants.

I wanted to share this to show that although changing your instincts is one of the hardest things you can endeavor to do, it *can* be done, and with effort, the rewards are immeasurable. So, it is only fitting that I will be dedicating the rest of my life to helping those who are still struggling or suffering with BPD. By writing this book and coaching with the FORDitude program that I have developed, I am happy to share some of the gifts of recovery that I have been blessed with.

Chapter 3

Navigating BPD Cover to Cover

"Courage is simply the willingness to be afraid and act anyway."

Robert Anthony

The *HOW* We Do It

This process is represented by the following essential key aspects: honesty, open-mindedness, and willingness. I learned the importance of these three necessary ingredients from the Alcoholics Anonymous program, and like most recipes, if you leave one of these ingredients out, the results will not be good.

Honesty

If you are not honest to and with yourself first, you will always have problems with not being able to trust yourself – and if you can't trust yourself, you won't have any quality of life, no matter what other efforts are made at self-improvement or development. I now call bullsh*t on myself and on anyone else who is still using the same old "stinking thinking" on that one.

If you are not honest with people in your life, including being dishonest by omission (my old favorite excuse as to why it was okay to not be 100 percent truthful – they didn't ask, so I did not feel I had to tell), then you are not to be trusted at all. And if you can't be trusted, what kind of friend are you or will you be?

Openminded

Are you able to have an open mind when confronted with new ideas that make you uncomfortable and likely fearful? We tend to instinctively fear those things that we don't have knowledge of or about. With fear there are always a couple of options: *F*** *E*verything *A*nd *R*un, or *F*ace *E*verything *A*nd *R*ecover. As I have shared elsewhere in this book, always look at your fear critically. As my psychologist, Larry, taught me to do, ask yourself the question "where is the evidence to support this thinking?" Another acronym for fear is *F*alse *E*vidence *A*ppearing *R*eal!

When we allow ourselves to be open to the possibilities, then truly incredible things can and will come into our lives. But if we are not open, they can't and won't. That is a fact.

Willingness

Are you willing to be willing? It is easier said than done, but thankfully, to be willing is really a state of mind – one determined by you. If you are willing to go to any lengths to recover your life and learn how to manage your mind, I can promise that you will be living a life that you only dreamt was possible. However, if you aren't willing to be willing, then you will have to be willing to settle for what you have had in the past. I believe that since you are still reading this book, you have decided you are willing to be willing. And that is amazing.

One tough question for you is this: are you willing to accept the fact that as part of your growth, you will have to become willing to sit with being uncomfortable? You must be willing to sit in your uncomfortable feelings, uncomfortable silences, and being uncomfortable period. You will learn through them that it becomes the way for you to be comfortable with your feelings, emotions, and silence. You will get a feeling of comfort in your skin and within yourself, and for some of us this will be the first time we have ever experienced this. I am willing to be willing, as I know the cost if I am not and the rewards if I am.

Willing to be Uncomfortable

A few weeks into working with Olivia, during a particularly difficult conversation, I had to literally put my hands up in a T for the universal time out sign to ask her to cease talking. She would ask me a question, and before I would get to the third word in my response, she would launch into a tirade about why she felt justified in wanting me to answer her question the way she wanted. I figured it wasn't a good use of our time or energy, and I was assertive the next time she did the same thing. She didn't like it and got quite frustrated with me. She proceeded to tell me, in a very defensive tone of voice, "I don't think that it's a good idea for us to continue talking about this. You obviously don't understand how I feel, and what I went through."

Although I did understand, I simply nodded my agreement to let her know that I heard and said nothing else. We both remained quiet for the next few minutes, and I could see her facial expressions changing, as though she was expecting me to resume the conversation and defend my position. When I didn't, she eventually looked up sheepishly and apologized for not allowing me to talk. Simply by refusing to engage with her and giving her a couple of minutes of sitting in an uncomfortable silence, she realized that it really was a one-sided conversation. At that point, we both had a little giggle and talked about it a bit further before concluding the session.

Healthier Lifestyle

Olivia had been struggling with working part-time as a server while attending university via distance learning to earn her social work degree. So, even though the effort required to get up and put one foot in front of the other every day is major, Olivia draws strength from the love she has for her daughter Rosie first, and then from her desire to change her life and get well. She has a willingness to do whatever it takes to learn how to manage her mind and her life in order to conquer BPD and to have a life she loves living. She has told me that she is already noticing positive changes in her thinking and in her behaviour since incorporating FORDitude into her life. Rosie is also benefiting from Olivia's improved mental health and overall well-being. Together they are more engaged in living a healthier lifestyle, which includes meal planning and fun with food purchases and preparation, a water drinking chart on their fridge complete with stars and hearts, a more consistent sleep schedule that benefits both mom and daughter, daily activities they take turns deciding on, and a few other activities that they are having fun doing together.

Building FORDitude

FORDitude came into existence as a daily action program, which I developed as the result of over a decade of lived experience and education in recovery from mental health and substance abuse issues. I have read hundreds of related books in my own recovery journey and have sourced and borrowed, with credit given, from a plethora of different areas and avenues. I have been influenced greatly by the foundational texts of AA and the Hazelden collections and works by experts such as Gabor Mate, Brene Brown, Melody Beattie, Louise Hay, Andrew Weil, Joseph Murphy, and Byron Katie, among countless others. I have attended many workshops and seminars over the last twenty plus years as well, ranging in topics related to my career in human resources and the financial sector to my more recent personal work in recovery from substance abuse and BPD. I have learned immeasurable lessons from years of dialectical behavioral therapy (DBT) and cognitive behavioral therapy (CBT) sessions, twelve-step meetings and step work, service work, volunteering, and treasured conversations with many wise souls over the years, both formally and non-formally educated.

Fortitude, according to the Merriam Webster Dictionary, is defined as follows: *the strength of mind that enables a person to encounter danger and bear pain or adversity with courage.* To me, this definition implies possessing two key characteristics: strength and resilience. From my experience with BPD, these were two characteristics I needed to grow within myself. By not having these characteristics developed, it would be a real hindrance to coping with the struggles of both daily life and managing my BPD. The ultimate inspiration and goal of this program is to help you learn and develop these essential characteristics as well. Backed by the skills and knowledge outlined in this book, I want to provide you the tools to develop the knowhow to create positive change in your life, overcome the barriers you feel and face as a result of your BPD, and build fortitude in your daily life. This is possible by understanding the reasons behind the steps of the program and practicing them daily.

Step 1 ~ Foundation of FORDitude

In the first step of FORDitude, I discuss the power of vulnerability, as discussed by Brene Brown in her book *Daring Greatly*. This way of thinking was very influential in building the FORDitude program, long before I even realized I was developing it.

Next, I explain the enormous benefits of viewing yourself as the ultimate project and of utilizing project management strategies to manage important aspects of your life.

You will learn to set realistic goals and timeframes in order to assist you with your ongoing life management. You will also learn how to do your own healing through effective time management, allowing you to focus on what is required to be able to perform to your highest good and provide for your body, mind, and spirit. In order to do this, I will show you how to organize your necessary tasks into steps which are actionable and accountable. Using the tool/table that I will share with you, I will show you how to lay out the day ahead and organize and sort out your "laundry list" of stuff to clear from your mind before sleep.

I will also go over why it is so important to ensure that you are consuming the appropriate amount of water daily and how to recognize signs of dehydration. Breathwork will be touched on here as well.

Step 2 ~ Optimize Your Mind and Spirit

In this step, I discuss the importance of beginning each day with positive intentions and reading daily meditations, Melody Beattie's "Language of Letting Go," as well as doing mirror work with positive affirmations.

I will walk you through the importance of knowing you can restart or reset your day anytime you want or need to. The option to "hit the reset button" and begin again with new intentions is always available to you. Yesterday is gone, tomorrow hasn't happened yet and today is a gift, which is why we call it the present. It is what we have, not all we have, and the key is to make the most of every day. Let's not waste a precious moment of our day looking backwards or forwards.

You can do anything for one day but having to think about doing it for the rest of your life can become too daunting a thought. Therefore, it is so important to live by the philosophy of "one day at a time."

Step 3 ~ Recognizing Your Resilience

In this step, you will learn about one man's story of how he gave his trauma a purpose, the three key qualities of resilience, what it is and whether you have to be born with it, or if you can learn it. You will learn more about the qualities of resilience and examples of how important they are day in and day out. Also, where thinking traps come from, why you may fall into them without even knowing they are there in the first place, and what, if anything, you can do to avoid them in the future.

We will explore other common issues you may be challenged with concerning limiting beliefs and unconscious thinking that you can become aware of and change once you become aware of, such as iceberg beliefs.

Step 4 ~ **Determine the Truth of the Matter**

In this step, you will learn about cooccurring disorders, addiction, and the definition and cause of addiction. I will introduce you to Canadian physician and four-time best-selling author Dr. Gabor Mate and his work in addiction and trauma, which has been instrumental to my personal recovery journey.

I will shed light on the stories we tell ourselves, which are full of negative self-talk, and what you can do to interrupt the inner dialogue that has been taking place in your head for a long time and replace it with a new one that is more suitable for you today.

Dependency in childhood and shame-based family systems that can contribute to your adverse childhood experiences will also be explored.

Step 5 ~ **Integrated Healing Approaches**

In this step, I will talk about several creative healing options to explore. The first thing to ensure is that you are getting enough sleep and that you are working on your conscious breathing, as both are extremely important to your day-to-day performance.

I will explore various art forms, like music and painting, and different forms of exercise, like yoga and qi gong. Next, I will discuss the many benefits of imagery and visualization and provide examples of each. Lastly, let's look at how important and helpful it is to establish a routine of expressive writing and journaling, including a daily gratitude exercise which will enable you to effectively deal with past issues that may still be causing you great challenges in your heart and mind.

Step 6 ~ Therapeutic Approaches (DBT & CBT)

In this step, I discuss that all therapy begins with awareness, our thoughts determine our future and we will discuss with you the avenues to pursue on your way to recovery from BPD, which include both Dialectic Behavioural Therapy (DBT) and Cognitive Behavioural Therapy (CBT), with a focus on mindfulness.

Step 7 ~ Universal Power and Connection to Recovery Supports

In this step, I will extend an invitation to you to connect to the "Source" of your understanding and choosing – be it the Universe, God (**G**ood **O**rderly **D**irection) or Goddess, Creator, Mother Nature, "That Which Pulls You Through," or any power greater than yourself. This a crucial piece that has been missing in Western medicine, and is known as the triangle of mind, body and spirit.

I will introduce the basics of Buddhism while emphasizing that spirituality, for me, has been the single best decision in helping me turn my life around.

I will discuss healthy connections, the value of pets and the unconditional love they bring into our lives, Buddhism as a form of more structured spirituality, several types of prayers, recovery supports, including online recovery groups, and the benefit of coaching.

Step 8 ~ **Depend on Yourself**

In this step, I will share a story from my early days of recovery, and a lesson that enough is enough in learning boundaries.

I will discuss how to understand the need and benefit of self-care, understanding what codependency is and what boundaries are. You will also learn about the role of appropriate anger, and how and why you will likely need to look at the key relationships in your life.

Lastly, I will outline the benefits of reducing/eliminating gluten and white sugar from your system and the cost to your physical and mental health if you don't because "you don't know, what you don't know."

Step 9 ~ **Elevate Yourself**

In this step, I will be sharing the key life-changing golden rules that I have picked up and adopted in my life and in my FORDitude Daily Action Program. Long before I developed the program that I used and integrated into my psyche, it became my moral compass in helping to make difficult decisions much easier as I followed these guidelines that are now second nature, like breathing – I don't even have to think about it anymore and it can take the guess work out of making decisions.

Obstacles and Conclusion

In the final two chapters, I will explore the benefits of moving forward and implementing the FORDitude Daily Action Program, the goals of doing so, and the huge costs associated with not doing the work, and therefore not getting the benefits in your 'New & Improved Life.' All the obstacles are surmountable *if* you want it bad enough and want your life to change. But remember, life doesn't get better by chance – but by change!

I won't pretend that this will be a cake walk because it won't be. It is your life that we are talking about, so it is worth the effort required and worth the time and the investment. There are no shortcuts in life to any place worth going, but the journey and the work will be so incredibly worth it. When you get to the place where the work and practice has paid off and you can see and notice it in your actions and your relationships, you will be blown away!

Chapter 4

Step 1

Foundation of FORDitude

"When we stop caring what people think, we lose our capacity for connection. When we become defined by what people think, we lose our willingness to be vulnerable."

Brene Brown

Vulnerability

In the introduction of this book and this program, I shared that I have taken great comfort and knowledge from the hundreds of books I have read during my recovery journey through BPD. One of the books that truly had an impact on my way of thinking was *Daring Greatly* by Brene Brown. In it she discusses her previous role as a shame researcher and shares that after she gave her first TED talk, she was cautioned not to read the comments, but she did so anyway. Many of the comments were not kind, and she was extremely hurt as a result. While she was trying to console herself afterwards, she came across a poem by Teddy Roosevelt that she claims changed her life. The poem is as follows:

> *"It is not the critic who counts; not the man who points out how the strong man stumbles, or where the doer of deeds could have done them better. The credit belongs to the man who is actually in the arena, whose face is marred by dust and sweat and*

blood; who strives valiantly; who errs, who comes up short again and again, because there is no effort without error and shortcoming; but who does actually strive to do the deeds; who knows great enthusiasms, the great devotions; who spends himself in a worthy cause; who at the best knows in the end the triumph of high achievement, and who at the worst, if he fails, at least fails while daring greatly, so that his place shall never be with those cold and timid souls who neither know victory nor defeat."

I have faced my own struggles with the willingness to be seen and to be vulnerable. Never professionally, as Brene Brown experienced and shared, but personally. In a professional context, I always managed to hide behind the mask I wore: my "human resources face" as I called it. I took such confidence from that role and its mask, and convinced myself that interacting with other professionals didn't bother me in the least. To have a personal conversation with someone was, for me, what took incredible courage and vulnerability that I often did not feel I had. It was incredibly difficult for me to show up and be seen for who I truly was because I truthfully did not know who that was. A large part of this struggle was the knowledge that my emotions were constantly unstable. All it took to turn me into a puddle of tears was a kind word or a look of genuine concern from someone around me.

If that sounds familiar, I am here to tell you that you can and will learn to manage your emotions with education, understanding, practice and reinforcement. I still marvel sometimes that I am able to keep my emotions and tears in check, but I can, more often than I ever imagined possible. I still tear up, but I have the tools and know-how to mindfully prevent a full-blown meltdown and that, my friend, is a feat I did not think would ever be possible for me. It takes a lot of hard work to learn to conquer the enormity of the swells of emotions, but conscious effort and reinforcement will prevail. As long as you do your part to manage your reactions to your circumstances and maintain a balanced approach to life, it is possible – one day at a time.

Project Management Skills for a Better Life

During a visit to my Grandma Ford's place several years ago, I had a conversation with my cousin Leo. He is a project manager for a big oil company in the tar sands. I remember saying to him that I marveled at how people hadn't caught on to the idea of using the concept and basis of project management for successfully managing their lives like businesses and companies have been doing for eons now. As a seasoned HR professional, in both the financial services sector and the IT contract staffing world, and an entrepreneur myself, I was very familiar with the principles of project management and why it worked so effectively to allow companies to succeed. Looking back now, I realize that conversation was a turning point for me, as I had already started implementing these ideas into my own life – though I didn't do it consciously at the time. I was newly sober then, and I was simply trying to do anything and everything I could to make my life simpler and more manageable. I have come to realize that I must have planted a seed in my subconscious that day, and thank goodness I did. It laid the foundation for the changes and growth I would experience in my life, not to mention the FORDitude Daily Action Plan program that I developed.

A Seed Is Planted and a Life Blooms

So, FORDitude all started with the simple idea that companies and businesses are much more likely to succeed if they have a few key things in place from the beginning. Why would it not make sense to think of ourselves, and our lives, as the *ultimate* project to manage? What asset could be more valuable than your own life? Certainly, none that I can think of. And how else will you know how to live your best life if you don't have the know-how and the tools as they are laid out in a business plan for instance?

What is a project? It is a temporary endeavor undertaken to create a unique product, service, or result. What better result could there be than a good life? A program is a recurrent project, which fits the description of what we will be doing: utilizing the program's steps on a daily basis to manage your most important tasks.

Some of the many benefits of using the Project Management philosophy are the following:

Better control over what you are doing and the expected outcome.

The ability to define your goals and determine what you will require to meet them.

Early knowledge of problems you may encounter, which will allow for corrective action.

Reduced stress and the ability to manage expectations more effectively – both yours and others.

Reliability and adaptability with information and knowledge.

Goal Setting Exercise

What goals and plans do you have the future?

- Goal Statement – write in one or two sentences.
- what needs to be accomplished and when it should be completed by?
- How you will know it is complete?
- Why is this goal important? And why is it worth accomplishing at this time?
- Explain how it will impact your life.
- What is needed to accomplish this goal? List the people, material, and equipment you will need to accomplish the goal.

Checklist to make sure your goal is well-defined.

SPECIFIC
- Is it clear what needs to be done to accomplish the goal?
- Is it clear who owns the goal and who you need to get support from to accomplish the goal? When completed by?

MEASURABLE
- Do you know how you will know when the goal has been completed?
- Does the goal statement indicate how many, how often, or how much?

ACHIEVABLE
- Do you feel you can achieve the goal by the target date?
- Do you feel you can get the support you need from others to accomplish the goal?
- Do you have access to all the material and equipment you need to accomplish the goal in the specified time period?

RELEVANT
- Is your goal going to improve your personal life?

TIME-BOUND
- Does your goal statement indicate when the goal needs to be completed?

ACTION PLAN – identify the key actions that need to be taken to complete your goal. Who and when and completed by what date?

GOAL LIST - Use this exercise format for each goal that you would like to set.

I use a spreadsheet for tracking my daily routine/activities; see the table below. However, you can begin by using a simple piece of paper on which you can keep track of a breakdown of necessary daily tasks. This will include a running list of new to-dos and carry forwards.

Time	Appointment	To-do
7:00 a.m.	Wake up and do conscious breathing	Read *Language of Letting Go* and set intentions for the day – mind work
7:30 a.m.	Hydrate with .5 litres of water and have nutritious breakfast	Coaching calls/reading/practicing
8:00 a.m.	Family/personal needs	
8:30 a.m.	Review yesterday's to-dos	
9:00 a.m.	Carry over any outstanding to-dos and create new ones for today	
9:30 a.m.		
10:00 a.m.	Active Engagement – daily activity of choice from Program List	
10:30 a.m.	Hydrate with .5 litres of water and have a healthy snack	**Errands**
11:00 a.m.	Expressive journaling exercise	Groceries/doctor appointments

Time	Appointment	To-do
11:30 a.m.		
12:00 p.m.	Hydrate with .5 litres of water and have nutritious lunch	
12:30 p.m.		
1:00 p.m.	Conscious breathing exercise and practice visualization or imagery	
1:30 p.m.		
2:00 p.m.	Read/watch a program to gain knowledge for skill improvement	Calls
2:30 p.m.		Schedule any appointments
3:00 p.m.	Hydrate with .5 litres of water and have a healthy snack	
3:30 p.m.		
4:00 p.m.	Domestic responsibilities – meal prep	

Time	Appointment	To-do
4:30 p.m.		
5:00 p.m.		
5:30 p.m.		
6:00 p.m.	Hydrate with .5 litres of water and have dinner	
6:30 p.m.	Family time or social activities/games	
7:00 p.m.		
7:30 p.m.		
8:00 p.m.	Connect with coach or supports i.e. call, zoom, email, etc.	
8:30 p.m.		
9:00 p.m.		
9:30 p.m.		

Time	Appointment	To-do
10:00 p.m.	Begin winding down with a warm bath, tea, quiet reflection and gratitude list	
10:30 p.m.		
11:00 p.m.	Rest for eight hours for much deserved and needed sleep – guided meditation	

Start each day by asking yourself a series of questions. First, what is on my plate today? Write it down and then ask, can I do anything about it? If you can't, write it down and give it to the Universe to hold for you, or put it in your burn pile. If you can, then write it on your to-do list. If there is an appointment you need to schedule, write it down, and it will be your reminder to call and schedule the appointment later in the day. You may want to print out your schedule for the day. Something I find helpful is specifying what actions and accountabilities I will need to outline. Later we will discuss in more detail exactly what you need to do, how to set goals to improve your ability to succeed, and how to accomplish what you have set out to do from one day to the next.

FORDitude Daily Action Program Components

Using FORDitude, you'll finally be able let go of the behaviours you had to learn and use to merely survive. There will be no need to hold onto them when you are thriving and no longer living in survival mode. You will establish new goals and attainable methods to achieve them and end up with new ideas and a new way of life.

Now it's time to put the program into action using your daily schedule and include the following items and ideas to make all aspects of your life easier to manage.

1. Make a list of all the things you are trying to juggle and prioritize daily/weekly/monthly.

2. Eliminate the unnecessary things that clutter your mind and your environment.

3. Ask for help from friends and family, and hire help if possible/needed to ease your burden. Don't be too shy to ask.

4. Combine activities such as calling your mom and doing laundry, or exercise and socializing; multi-task whenever possible to minimize time spent on tasks.

5. Use the KISS principle (Keep It Simple Sweetheart), and simplify all that you can, from doing all the shopping on one day or arranging to get it delivered. Keep activities close to home and schedule them only over two days, not all seven days of the week.

6. Eliminate/minimize distractions and time drains such as email and social media.

7. Work efficiently by visualizing what you need to get done and making a to-do list. This helps you identify all of the "mission critical" items you need for the day, and at the end of the day, carry forward any that weren't completed to the next day. If there is something on your mind, but there is nothing that you can do about it now, write it down and put it in your "Let It Go" Box, so it can be taken back out when you are able to take action on it, but not until then.

8. Work with your preferences. If you are a morning person, do the things that require the most effort first thing. Likewise, if having too much scheduled makes you feel trapped, stick with daily and weekly to-do lists.

9. Remember to "sharpen the saw." It takes much longer to cut something with a dull saw. When you don't get enough sleep and recreation, you may start to feel unbalanced in your life.

Taking Inventory

As with any business conducting a regular inventory, to "take stock" be accountable, look for expired/unsalable products/goods, it makes sense for us to do the same process personally, and be willing to take an honest moral inventory of ourselves so that we may begin to look the in some of following areas:

How do I think of myself?

How do I see my relationships with other people?

What is my general sense of personal well being?

What fears do I have about the future?

What resentments do I have about the past?

What is the cause for these resentments?

How do these past resentments affect my current self?

What can I do to move past these past resentments?

What emotions do I feel now? Are these valid?

Getting Clear on Priorities

It is easy to distract ourselves with stuff that fills up our days and adds nothing of any real value to our lives. It is important to resist the urge to do this by not adding to your schedule the activities and events that don't reflect your values and top priorities. When you're struggling to find the time for the big ones, like ensuring you have adequate sleep, make use of the evolving daily list of what's most important, and you will soon see how you spend your days and how much time you are dedicating to those things.

Feeling as Good as You Can: Progressive Physician

I had been slightly to moderately overweight most of my adult life, with a five-foot-six-inch frame. What that really means is this: there had been a few periods of my life that I had been in great shape, but those days were long ago. I was eating to console my feelings, and my stomach was always tender and sore. I had ongoing issues with constipation and diarrhea, seemingly always dealing with one or the other, and never knowing what it was like to have a "regular" bowel movement. I had to take medications to counteract the acid reflux and other effects that my daily medications had on the lining of my stomach. It seemed my tummy was always bloated, and it literally hurt to put any pressure on it whatsoever.

Thankfully, I began to see a Doctor who was very forward-thinking, and she suggested that an important area for me to consider was food sensitivities. She recommended that I see a naturopathic doctor in Victoria, a city three hours away from where I live on Vancouver Island, British Columbia. I had a series of tests including food allergies, metals and adrenal.

Water Consumption and Dehydration

One of the things that I learned from ND was how important water is. We humans are largely made up of water, and it is vitally important that we drink enough daily to ensure that we can perform all bodily tasks properly. On average for men, that is 3 liters a day, and for women, 2.2 liters a day.

What does water do for you? It forms saliva needed for digestion, keeps mucosal membranes moist, and it allows the body's cells to grow, reproduce, and survive. It also flushes body waste, mainly in urine, and it lubricates joints. Water is a major component of most body parts and is needed to manufacture hormones and neurotransmitters, regulate body temperature through sweating and respiration, acts as a shock absorber for the brain and spinal column, convert food components needed for survival through the digestion process, and help deliver oxygen all over the body.

Foundation – How Do You Build a House?

If you have spent any time on a construction site, you may know that before any of the actual structural components are built, the concrete foundation is constructed and poured. Well, that's the same concept that we are discussing here. Before we can look at beginning construction on the top floor of the house, we have to ensure that the foundation is secure and has been poured properly. Once that step has been completed and the cement has had time to cure, the carpenters can come back to the job site and begin framing the rest of the building and attach it securely to the foundation and the footings. They know it will be safe and will be secure in the fact that the house won't come tumbling down on top of them, because it is fastened to and anchored into the ground.

Building the foundation for FORDitude was constructed with the same concern and care. I used my common sense when building the program and added the knowledge and skills that I believe are necessary for success. I added examples from my life and those of others who I have coached to illustrate what I am explaining and teaching, and I also added humor to make the learning a little more enjoyable.

Chapter 5

Step 2

Optimize Your Mind and Spirit

"Today, God, help me not judge or limit my future by my past. Help me be open to all the exciting possibilities for change, both within and around me."

Melody Beattie

One Day at a Time
Is the Magical Way to Life Your Life

"One day at a time" sounds more manageable than thinking about doing something for the rest of your life – right? Thinking of it that way makes it seem possible because it is! We *can* do anything for just twenty-four hours, but to think of never doing something *ever* again is so overwhelming that it can cause you to stop starting before you even consider starting. Confused? I know I was! I could not even contemplate the idea of not doing something, no matter what it was, for the rest of my life. And I had huge resistance to that idea! From the Law of Attraction, I also know that what we resist persists, so that was not going to make the daily struggle to stay stopped any easier until I found a better way to think about what I could do.

The concept of taking things just one day at a time works in so many ways, and the songs written about it are further proof of that. It is simple, and so effective.

Another trick to help establish your new way of thinking is knowing that you can break the time down into smaller chunks of time – one hour or even one minute – until you are comfortable and feel good about the fact that you *can* do what you put your mind to. As you build both your successes and your confidence, your successful days will accumulate, and before long, you will have time under your belt, and you will start to see changes in yourself and your behaviours. The more time you accumulate, the more confidence you will acquire, and the easier it will become.

How I Start Each Day

I was very fortunate many years ago to have a close friend of mine share a gift with me. The gift was introducing me to an author and a book that would have a huge impact on my life and my understanding of relationships, especially the one with myself – the relationship I understood the least. As you'll recall when I spoke of the impact that books have had on my healing journey, one of my favorite authors, Melody Beattie, wrote a book that left me wanting to learn more from her, and I had to read more. I found and fell in love with her daily meditation book, which I read at the start of everyday, and I always feel better for having read it. I can't imagine starting my day without the guidance and inspiration that it provides for me daily.

Melody Beattie integrates her own life experiences and fundamental recovery reflections in this unique daily medi-ation book, which she wrote especially for those of us who struggle with the issue of codependency. Melody Beattie reminds us that problems are made to be solved, and the best thing we can do is take responsibility for our own pain and self-care. Each day she writes on different topics that we face and weaves in life situations and solutions, with a focus on self-empowerment and spirituality.

I would encourage you to also start each day by reading *The Language of Letting Go* by Melody Beattie to begin your day on the right foot. I would like to share with you today's meditation as an incredible example of a powerful reading, and why I decided many years ago after becoming aware of her through her book *Codependent No More*, to begin each day with reading her material.

Melody Beattie's Daily Meditations for Codependency Language of Letting Go

You Are Not a Victim

How deeply engrained your self-image as a victim can be! How habitual your feelings of misery and helplessness! Victimization can be like a grey cloak that surrounds us, both attracting that which will victimize you and cause you to generate feelings of victimization. Victimization can be so habitual that you may feel victimized even by the good things that happen to you!

I have learned that if you set your mind to it, you have an incredible, almost awesome, ability to find misery in any situation, even the most wonderful of circumstances.

Shoulders bent, head down, you shuffle through life taking your blows.

Be done with it. Take off the gray cloak of despair, negativity, and victimization. Hurl it; let it blow away in the wind.

You are not a victim. You may have been victimized. You may have allowed yourself to be victimized. You may have sought out, created, or recreated situations that victimized you, but you are not a victim. You can stand in your power. You do not have to allow yourself to be victimized. You do not have to allow others to victimize you. You do not have to seek out misery in either the most miserable or the best situations. You are free to stand in the glow of self-responsibility.

Set a boundary! Deal with the anger! Tell someone no or stop that! Walk away from a relationship! Ask for what you need! Make choices and take responsibility for them! Explore options. Give yourself what you need and stand up straight, head up, and claim your power. Claim responsibility for yourself! And learn to enjoy what is good!

Today, I will refuse to think, talk, speak, or act like a victim. Instead, I will joyfully claim responsibility for myself and focus on what is good and right in my life.

You Can Heal Your Life

It was through the amazing work that Louise Hay has done, which I learned about in her book *You Can Heal Your Life*, that I began to understand the what, how and why of affirmations.

In her book *You Can Heal Your Life*, Louise Hay shares her belief that as you grow from the perfection of a baby into the problems of an adult, it is because you felt unworthy and unlovable to some degree. This is due to limiting beliefs which you were raised with that were passed down from parents and caregivers. I know it took me a long time to be able to move from a place of blame to a place of understanding, and that has enabled me to rise above the issues of my past and make positive changes in my future.

I learned that in order to fully understand my childhood, first I had to know what had happened to both of my parents before the age of ten to even begin to imagine what it must have been like for them growing up. What kind of childhood would have created an adult like that? And furthermore, I would need this knowledge for my own freedom. I began to realize that I couldn't forgive myself until I could forgive them first.

I also learned to "examine my thoughts" and the notion that whatever we believe will come true, which was a huge discovery for my recovery. I have learned to ask myself questions concerning my thoughts to determine if they are appropriate for me today. I now ask myself, "Is it true for me now?" and "Would I be better off if I dropped that belief?" These questions help me to let go of old limiting beliefs that no longer serve me well. I will discuss more about limiting beliefs, specifically iceberg beliefs and how they impact your unconscious thinking, in Step 3.

Louise Hay states, "as you learn to control your mind by the conscious choice of thoughts, you align yourself with the incredible power that is intelligence that is within you constantly responding to thoughts and words." As you begin to consciously change your thoughts, when the old ones return, say to your mind, "I now choose to believe it is easier for me to make changes." And remember that the only thing that can be controlled is your current thought.

A very important daily practice of mine comes directly from this book and Louise Hay's teachings about affirmations. Knowing that what you focus your attention on grows is the basis for how affirmations works in our lives. Affirmations are positive statements that are made about what you want to have in your life. These are not just verbal statements. How you think about yourself and your life and are equally as important as what you say aloud. The goal of an affirmation is to open a channel in your consciousness to create what you have affirmed. Continually make positive statements about how you want your life to be, and be sure to state it in the present tense. For instance, "I am", or "I have". Your subconscious mind is so obedient that if you declare in the future tense "I want" or "I will have," then that is where it will stay – out of your reach!

Daily Positive Affirmations

When possible, look in a mirror and read these important messages to yourself daily until they become a part of your programming. The goal is not to memorize them but practice them daily to help imprint new pathways in your brain. It will improve how you feel about yourself, and help you begin acting "as if", until you can believe that you *are*.

- I am a caring and considerate person, always doing the best I can and always growing in wisdom and love.
- I am able to manage my thoughts and, as a result, my own life.
- My number one goal and personal responsibility is my own growth and well-being.
- I am compassionate and gentle with myself, therefore, I am gentler and more compassionate with others.
- I make my own good decisions and take full responsibility of my actions.
- My personal well-being depends on my attitude and acceptance, and it does not mean I approve of what has happened.
- I do not have to prove myself to anyone. I need only express myself as honestly and effectively as I am capable.
- My emotional well-being is dependent primarily on how I love me and how well I take care of my needs.
- I live one day at a time and do first things first.
- I am willing to be patient with myself today, for I have the rest of my life in which to grow and develop.
- Each experience I have in life contributes to my learning and growth.

Sarah's Magical Life

Like magic, changes happen, and one day you wake up and feel different. Sarah laughed as she told me about the first time she realized that she was embracing living her life "one day at a time". She had always been in a rush to do everything and wasted most of her time. But once Sarah embraced the Daily Action Program idea and had been working at it for a couple of weeks, she quickly began to notice that things in her day seemed to go much easier for her. Since using the FORDitude agenda to manage them, no longer did she find she was taking her medications late or missing them altogether. She was no longer running back and forth between her office at home and the downtown office as much as before because she was staying on track more and prioritizing her day in advance. Her productivity levels increased during the day, and she was getting more efficient scheduling appointments and client sessions with time available to focus on self-care. I could see in her face during our next session how relaxed she was, and her huge smile was from ear to ear. It was also great to hear her sound so positive when talking about her future plans.

Yesterday is history. Tomorrow is a mystery. Today is a present. Life is magic when you believe it.

Chapter 6

Step 3

Recognizing Your Resilience

"Proactively working to develop mental strength increases your resilience to stress and reduces the toll it takes on you both physically and mentally."

Amy Morin

Trauma and Resiliency

Instead of watching cable TV, I spend my free time watching and learning from TED talks. It never ceases to amaze me that an average person can get up on stage, share a part of their life with us, and not only do we hear some of our own story in theirs, but we can be so impacted by their experience and truth.

One evening while exploring on the topic of resilience, I came across, "What Trauma Taught Me About Resiliency," by Charles Hunt. He tells his story of giving his trauma purpose by surviving and succeeding despite having a drug addicted mother and a father who was a pimp and felon. Charles talks about his life especially from the ages of 7 to 10, during which he experienced several traumatic events, and what those experiences taught him. Most especially, finding his mother's boyfriend dead from a drug overdose, laying on the floor, and seeing the word "incarcerated" for the first time, on a letter he received from his father who was in jail. Then later, when he was called and informed that his father was brain dead from a prison fight, he had been in earlier that day. The pain, shame, and sadness he felt when his mother was also imprisoned was massive, but he decided that although he had been through some awful things in his life, he wouldn't let them get the best of him.

Charles would go on to graduate and earn his master's degree and become very successful personally as well as in the corporate world, because he knew the only thing constant is change. He had the ability to adapt and recover from negative and hurtful things. He chose to respond instead of reacting, to surmount obstacles instead of succumbing to them, and to work to understand how his early experiences impacted his beliefs, which affected his feelings about himself. Then how thoughts impact feelings, which then determine how he must respond. He was able to escape the hell he was living in by believing that tomorrow would somehow be better than today, and somehow, he knew to use the most powerful resource he had, the one we all have: his mind. He used his mind's power to overcome and succeed, and when you use that tool with the proper perspective and the proper attitude you can do anything, especially when you are able to ask others for help. Also, by acknowledging that we have been victims but then refuse to own it, we have the power to overcome anything believing it happens for a reason.

So, let's be thankful our trauma has a purpose and that is in helping us to see our strength to overcome it. It goes back to the reason that I decided to write this book – that by telling my story, it could be someone else's survival guide.

Three Keys of Resiliency

First, you will have to begin by accepting what is or has happened as it is and acknowledge the situation is simply part of life – but that doesn't mean you have to like it as it currently is.

Second, we use selective attention with a focus on the things you can affect change on or with. This includes identifying things you were grateful for in any situation. Regardless of the outcome, remember there is always something we can choose to be thankful about, and you can also choose to put your focus on the positive aspects of any situation.

Last, no matter the situation at hand, ask yourself the question, "is what you are doing helping you or harming you?" Is the situation manageable? Are you being kind to yourself? Reasonable? Realistic?

What Is Resilience and Why Is It So Important?

There are many definitions of resilience, and they often vary between different cultures and situations, but it generally refers to a person's ability to "cope well with adversity" and "persevere and adapt when things go awry." Resilient people are better able to deal with stress, adversity, overcome childhood disadvantages, and take on new opportunities. The way we think about stress is very much in our control and makes a big difference in how we handle daily bumps in the road. Some people feel helpless in the face of stress and adversity, so they give up attempting to change or improve the situation. Others see situations as challenges or problems that can be solved if they look for options and keep trying.

A resilient view is characterized by accurate and flexible thinking, creative problem-solving, the capacity to see other points of view and to adjust one's own views, and the ability to move on with daily life despite the obstacles.

Resilient Thinking Can Be Learned

Being resilient is important because it is a thread that runs through all aspects of our lives. Adverse events can endanger our development, health, or happiness all along our lifespan and making our way through such threats is vital. Understanding how one keeps their feet planted on the ground in the face of a threat is necessary because it allows us to better assist individuals to develop internal and external assets and supports that will help those individuals overcome adversity.

If you can view adversity or "bumps in the road" as a challenge instead of a huge disruption to your life, you will be more likely to thrive in whatever you do and handle stress with more ease.

Some people seem to have a natural disposition or temperament that lays a foundation for resiliency, which is a pattern of response. It is not something that one is born with. In a manner of speaking, it is not something that one "is", "has", or "doesn't have." The literature on the subject now views the nature of resilience and human development as a complex interaction between many levels of the individual and the environment.

The basic abilities that contribute to resilience can be developed through a process found in normal human

development, and the continued development of these
abilities will help you respond well throughout your life.

Qualities of Resilience

Belonging

Belonging is the feeling of being a part of something larger
than yourself. It is the feeling of belonging to a family, a
network of friends, a country, or a community. When people
feel they belong, it can lead to a more positive sense of self
and make it easier to participate in society and be successful.

I feel I belong when...a stranger smiles at me on the street
- or - l welcomed and accepted for who I am.

Emotional Regulation

Emotional regulation is being in charge of your emotions
enough to stay calm under pressure and being able to
express your emotions in ways that will help rather than
hurt a situation.

I know I am emotionally regulating when...I am able to
take three deep breaths before reacting when I am angry
or upset - or - I am aware of strong emotions as they arise,
and I don't get swept away by them.

Impulse Control

Impulse control is the ability to stop and choose whether to
act on a desire. For example, when you are angry and you
want to shout and argue, but instead you stop, back up, and
think about what would help the situation.

I know I am practicing impulse control when...I am able to use words to express my emotions - or - I am able to see when I'm getting worked up, think about why I'm upset, and then figure out what I can do about it.

Casual Analysis

Casual analysis is the ability to analyze a problem, accurately decide what its cause is, and be able to take a step back and assess a situation objectively.

I know I'm practicing causal analysis when...I feel clear and at least relatively calm about a situation, not confused and out of control - or - I am able to turn "I never" into "I didn't this time, but I will next time" thinking.

Realistic Optimism

Realistic optimism is the ability to maintain the belief that a brighter future is possible. This is not about seeing only the positive things in life and turning a blind eye to the negative, but about seeing things as they are and working at creating the future you want to have.

I know I am practicing realistic optimism when...I am able to see my successes even if I struggle or fail sometimes - or - I recognize my feelings of frustration, disappointment, or what have you, but I don't let those rule me and after I've rested, I move forward again.

Empathy

Empathy is the ability to understand the feelings and needs of another person and "walk in their shoes".

I know I am practicing empathy when...I am able to understand the feelings and needs of someone else - or - I recognize that others are different from me and might see and feel things differently than I do.

Self-Efficacy

Self-efficacy is the feeling of being effective in the world, making a difference, and having an impact. It is the belief that what you do matters. Self-efficacy is rooted in actual experience. When you are given opportunities to choose and to succeed based on those choices, you are more likely to have a sense of self-efficacy.

I know I'm practicing self-efficacy when...I feel as though I have what it takes to tackle problems and bounce back from them - or - I believe that what I do day-to-day matters.

Reaching Out

Reaching out is the ability to take on new opportunities that life presents, see things as learning opportunities, and take a risk sometimes. Reaching out is also about how much you can cope with and your ability to ask for help when you need it.

I know I'm reaching out when...I continue trying even when I make mistakes, and I understand that a mistake is not a failure when I have learned from it - or - I know myself and know how much I can handle, and I am not afraid of asking for help when I need it.

Language and Culture

Language and culture are having a connection to your language and culture of choice. For indigenous people, and in many other ethnic communities, being able to speak your traditional language and live according to cultural traditions is fundamental to resilience.

When it comes to language and culture...

- It can be much harder for the other qualities to take root without this basic ground
- For the indigenous people's resiliency, it includes healing from negative experiences, such as residential school, and reclaiming their language and culture as individuals and as a society in relation to a larger settler nation that continues at times to act as if indigenous people are "in the way"
- Culture of choice isn't always culture of birth; For example, women born into a culture that restricts their freedom may feel more comfortable in a different culture

Response to Stress and Adversity
The Three P's

Patterns and explanatory styles that we develop when reacting to stress and adversity are our ways of viewing what is happening in the world. This makes it more difficult for us to think flexibly and accurately about a situation.

Dr. Martin Seligman from the University of Pennsylvania has studied resilience for more than three decades now and his findings have led to the following results. He found that how people explain their success and failures influences whether they preserve or give up when faced with adversity. The research shows that people unconsciously look for answers to three questions when trying to make sense of what happened to them.

They are:

1. **Personalization:** Who caused the problem?
   (Me/Not me)
2. **Permanence:** How long will this problem last?
   (Always/Not always)
3. **Pervasiveness:** How much of my life does this problem affect? (Everything/Not everything)

The important thing about the explanatory style is that it causes us to react out of habit and jump to conclusions that may not be accurate. This prevents us from using the kind of flexible thinking that promotes problem solving and leads to positive change.

Thinking Habits Associated with Depression, Aggression, and Optimism

I can remember back to a client I worked with named Beth. She would describe feeling like she was such as loser, she'd never get the "girl", and nobody likes her. This description is typical of "Me/Always/Everything" thinking – an explanatory pattern related to "pessimistic" thinking. This kind of thinking can lead to a loss of hope and to depression among people who get in the habit of using it. With "Me" statements like "I am such a loser", Beth takes the situation personally and blames herself. It is also an example of "Always" and "Everything" thinking: If she really thinks all this is true, there is no way for Beth to make her life better. Even if she's just feeling frustrated, thinking like that isn't helpful and will just make her feel worse.

"Not me/Always/Everything" thinking can also be a problem and tends to result in blaming others when something bad happens and experiencing a sense of futility when things go wrong. This thinking, instead of leading to depression, can make people feel trapped and angry, or cause them to lash out at others.

While a "Not me/Not always/Not everything" thinking style may be the most optimistic explanatory style, it may not be an accurate or very realistic view of a situation. People who use this style in all situations run the risk of losing out on genuine relationships since their cheerful outlook might ignore difficult issues that exist between themselves and others. The goal is to maintain realistic optimism by thinking as accurately and flexibly as possible about each situation you face.

Thinking Traps

Dr. David Burns wrote the book *Feeling Good: The New Mood Therapy*, and was the first to capture and compile the information regarding the mental shortcuts we take to simplify the information our brains take in, using our five senses to assist in the process. Especially in times of stress, these shortcuts are automatic and largely unconscious. Because they can trap us into drawing conclusions prematurely, they have been called thinking traps.

Most people have a strong bias when they process information. We tend to use only the information that supports the beliefs we already have about a situation and we filter out information that does not support our beliefs. This is called confirmation bias. It can stop us from using accurate and flexible thinking to assess situations, causing us to draw conclusions with less information than we, ideally, need.

Common Thinking Traps

- **Jumping to conclusions**: making assumptions about people or situations with little or no evidence to back it up.
- **Personalizing**: assuming blame for problems or situations for which you are not primarily responsible
- **Externalizing**: blaming others for situations for which they are not primarily responsible
- **Mindreading**: assuming you know what others are thinking without checking with them or expecting others to know what you are thinking without telling them
- **Emotional reasoning**: making false conclusions about an experience based on how you feel rather than on the facts
- **Overgeneralizing**: making sweeping judgements about someone or something based on only one or two experiences
- **Magnifying/minimizing**: over emphasizing certain aspects of a situation and shrinking the importance of other aspects
- **Catastrophizing**: assuming something bad is going to happen or exaggerating how bad a situation will be

Iceberg Beliefs

Some beliefs are difficult to identify because they are deeper and more complex. Identifying them or at least becoming aware of them is one key to being resilient. These beliefs operate mostly on the subconscious level, lying like icebergs beneath the surface, and are powerful forces that can significantly undermine your resilience and your relationships. Iceberg beliefs can cause extremely intense reactions that take you by surprise and may seem out of proportion to actual situations. These beliefs start to form in childhood and are often passed down unconsciously, without question, from generation to generation. Family transmitted iceberg beliefs like "Never let them know you are hurting" or "boys shouldn't cry" could prevent a people from reaching out to others for help. They have deeply rooted beliefs about how the world should operate and how they should operate in the world. These deeply rooted beliefs could look like:

"I should be able to handle anything that comes my way."

"Women should never show their anger."

"People should always be on time."

Iceberg beliefs can make us over experience certain emotions. For example, the belief "things should always be fair' could lead you to overreact to the many inequities that are bound to happen in daily life.

Iceberg beliefs can be at the root of personality clashes. For instance, if one person believes "it's important to be liked by everyone," that person may not express any opinions that might be unpopular. A person who believes "it's important that people express their opinions," may challenge others and be seen as argumentative.

Not all iceberg beliefs cause negative outcomes. Many of our values are based on iceberg beliefs, and they can motivate us to maintain positive relationships, resolve conflicts, and make use of opportunities that come our way. These positive beliefs could look like:

"Mistakes are a part of learning process"

"Honesty is the best policy"

"If you don't succeed at first, try again"

Types of Iceberg Beliefs

- **Achievement**: People who have these type of iceberg beliefs see success as the most important thing in life and often see mistakes as failures. The expectation is perfection, they will feel anxious about their performance or become highly critical of others' contributions.

- **Acceptance**: This is the idea that it's vital to be liked, accepted, praised, and included by others. These type iceberg beliefs tend to make people blame themselves for situations or act in ways that make them feel bad later.

- **Control**: People who have these type of iceberg beliefs have unrealistic expectations about the level of influence they have over themselves and their environment. They become uncomfortable when circumstances are out of their direct control. Sometimes they will act in negative ways to try and gain control back – most times with unfavorable results.

Detecting Your Iceberg Beliefs

While working with Sarah, one of the main areas that she wanted to focus on was identifying her iceberg beliefs. As I explained to her, the process begins with awareness, as it does with most behaviours, and being able to recognize that a belief is "in play" and understanding that your reaction is out of proportion with what happened. Are you finding yourself being rigid about something without really understanding why? Are you are getting feedback from several people that you are being ridiculous? Do you feel paralyzed by a decision you are in the middle of making? Does it feel like there's a rule you need to follow or a moral issue?

In order to process further, if any of the above are true, ask the following questions next:

- What is the belief underneath my reaction?
- Is the belief accurate? Is it important to me?
- Is it just a case of one idea vs. another?
- What does the belief mean to me?
- Should I replace the belief with something else? What would happen if I did?

This process of asking one question after another helps to chip away at frozen, inflexible beliefs so you can begin to see beneath the surface of your reactions. This thawing, or melting, done slowly is more effective as well because it gives you an opportunity to make the change gradually.

With greater impact and improved awareness, this improves the overall success rate of repeating the new questioning behaviors so you can further chip away and melt into a new and better set of beliefs that will serve you more appropriately at this stage and age in your life.

Chapter 7

Step 4

Determining the Truth of the Matter

"The capacity of young people to persevere, even under the most adverse conditions, never ceases to amaze me."

Jane Fonda

My Alcoholism and BPD

I began drinking at the age of eight, but it wasn't like I had it planned that way – it just kind of happened. Sheri, my slightly older cousin, lived in the big city of Halifax, Nova Scotia, and I lived in the much smaller Annapolis Valley, 150 kilometers away. I am not sure what the occasion was on that particular trip into the big city, but I remember that all the "adults" were upstairs at Auntie Marilyn's split level house, and Sheri and I were downstairs on the pull out couch with our first drink in hand, beer and tomato juice mixed in a glass so if someone came down and saw us they'd be none the wiser. We loved that Sheri's mom, my mom's older sister, owned a restaurant and bar in the city because that meant that the bar, complete with mirrors and a full-size fridge in her rec room, was stocked full of many types of liquor. We were so excited and decided that we were going to sample each and every one of the bottles that night – and we almost succeeded.

We got very drunk and it is a wonder that neither one of us ended up with alcohol poisoning or more sick than we were, but sick we were, and back in those days, it was enough of a lesson that "your hangover will teach you not to do that again". When they found me, I was in the bathroom, on the floor, passed out, lying in a puddle of vomit. Suffice it to say, it would not be the last time I ended up in that exact same position – just different bathrooms.

It would be another thirty years before I would find the courage to walk into recovery for alcoholism. I started that journey ten years ago, and it has been far from a smooth ride. A year after my first foray into sobriety, I was diagnosed with borderline personality disorder, at thirty-nine years of age. I was still sober, but completely insane, or so I thought, with no higher power or viable coping skills for my out of control and volatile emotions. I was circling the drain and ready to commit suicide, and yet, even "failing" at that.

I was very fortunate to have been working with an amazing sponsor, Marie, who was a long-time family friend that I knew well. She had a psychology background and literally showed up and loved me until I began to love myself. She taught me the basics of how to start my day, important questions to ask, and how to assign importance to my list of things to do, or if I should "give it to God for now". She helped me to develop and embrace spirituality. In fact, in the beginning, she "loaned' me her higher power until I was able to believe in one of my own. That gift was priceless and really did change my life.

With her help and support, I was able to eventually put in place an action program for living that works for me, but most importantly, I was able to finally fill the hole that I had felt in my soul with my own conception of my Creator. My addiction to alcohol is/was a symptom of the bigger issue for me, which is that of lack of connection and feeling like I didn't fit it. I didn't even know who I was to begin with. In one incredible video about BPD on YouTube, which I would encourage everyone to watch (called "Back from the Edge"), Marsha Linehan describes BPD as the "I don't fit in" disorder. Boy, did that really resonate with me.

I realize now how much I relied on many different addictions over the years to provide relief from the pain I was feeling. It was my attempt to fill the void or the hole that I felt in my soul, but the truth of the matter is, the only thing that feels right, good, and just in filling that space is my spirituality. No temporary sensation, no food, clothing, substance, or behavior is going to ever provide that sense of fulfillment. I will continue to build and enjoy that for the remaining moments and days of my life.

Thankfully, I was able to find my sobriety, although, not easily. As it is said, and I have said earlier, please keep coming back and don't give up on you, until your miracle happens. Thank goodness I didn't, because it really did happen for me!

Definition of Addiction

Dr. Mate, defines addiction as "any behaviour in which the individual finds temporary pleasure in and craves for that reason – despite negative consequences." He goes on to say, "addictive behaviour can take on many forms and certainly is not limited to substance use." People can become addicted to shopping, sex, food, or any behaviour that they find brings feelings of pleasure. They are looking for temporary fulfilment – no matter the consequences. Mate has written four bestselling books on topics that range from attention deficit disorder in *Scattered Minds*, addiction and mental health issues in *In the Realm of Hungry Ghosts*, and the connection between mind, body, and spirit in *When the Body Says No*.

Mate was born in Nazi-occupied Budapest, Hungary in 1944, and he has shared that his young, Jewish mother was not able to meet his needs as a baby. Not because she did not love her young son, but because she was dealing with such fear and anxiety existing in those conditions. Dr. Mate realized that he learned at a very early age to disconnect and employ maladaptive coping strategies in order to be able to self-soothe in the absence of love and attachment from his mother, which all infants have an innate need for. He discovered that he had ADD in his 50s, and subsequently challenged the definition of the condition as a disease. He suggested, instead, that ADD is a coping skill of "tuning out", which is carried forward from infancy or childhood, and that this is the cause of the condition.

One of Mate's most powerful speeches that I have watched was at a recent conference in Scotland, called ACEs (Adverse Childhood Experiences) to Assets, where he was the keynote speaker. There, he discussed at length his career working in the medical field and that, in his opinion, trauma is the root cause of most addiction issues.

Dr. Mate believes that parents do their best raising their kids based on the role models and examples they had when they were being raised. However, as parents, we are only able to teach our children what we have learned ourselves;

therefore, it stands to reason that many children born of parents that were traumatized will lack fundamental skills to subsequently transfer to their children.

Adverse childhood experience (ACE) screenings allow medical professionals to assess children and determine the likelihood of future medical issues and cognitive challenges due to the environmental factors that affected how the child was raised. It is an incredibly accurate predictor, and it shows the relationship as far back as when the mother was carrying the fetus in utero as to the significance of stress hormones and how it influences the baby.

Testing was done with mothers and their babies that were born following the tragic events on 9/11, and there is evidence to support a definite correlation between the amount of stress that the mother was under while pregnant and the impact of the medical conditions present in their children. Learning difficulties, addiction issues, etc. were found to be directly related to the stress experienced by these children's mothers during the terrorist attacks.

Other studies conducted at the University of Washington in Seattle have determined the stress levels of moms during pregnancy can be measured in their babies at six months of age. That is incredible and so scary when you think about it, but it really supports what I have personally believed for a long time. It has never been a question of whether the parents love their children, it is whether the parents are equipped with the right skills and tolerance for managing a new baby effectively. As any parent out there knows, babies do not arrive with an instruction manual, unfortunately, and we all do our best to figure it out as we go.

Causes of Addiction

In one of Dr. Mate's articles, "A New Understanding of Addiction," he states that the belief is the root cause of addiction and the loss or of lack of connection to family, relationships, culture, spirituality, work, or any other important area in your life. He goes on to state that he believes that addiction is a disease, although it is much too large to fit the narrow confines of the disease model. Therefore, based on his research and over a decade of my own personal experience working with people in recovery, it is an individual's inability to deal with pain from early childhood experiences, including trauma, that results in addictive behaviours to numb and attempt to block the pain.

Even when these early experiences do not warrant the person feeling shame, as that person is an innocent victim, it most often is accompanied by fear. Addicts will reach for the only perceived control they know – external control to alter their feelings and mood in order to temporarily feel better as they had not developed coping mechanisms as children. This very confusing pattern will continue for the addict, until the very nature of addiction can be explained and eventually understood if the addict has the capacity to do so. This becomes much more difficult and complicated when the addict presents cooccurring disorders as discussed in this chapter.

During his time working in the lower East Side of Vancouver, British Columbia, Dr. Mate reports that every woman he treated for addiction had been sexually abused previously in their lives. They did not volunteer this information to him willingly, but during appointments and examinations, he would talk to and gather history and uncover this fact. As interesting was the knowledge that in a lot of situations, the women thought they were to blame and were bad – contrary to the supporting evidence. More broadly, but no less importantly, it needs to be said that Dr. Mate believes that all addicts have experienced trauma, but not all who experience traumatic events in their lives will become addicts.

Addiction May be Part of Your Story

For those of us who have live with BPD, it is not surprising when addiction is also part of your story. There is a desire to block out the pain, be it emotional, mental, or physical. It is especially hard for those nonaddict types who can have one or two of whatever it is to understand why we can't just stop after one. I would always say that for me, "One was too many, and twenty wasn't enough", and nothing could have described my addictive personality better. As an alcoholic, I would eventually get to the end goal, the point of no more pain, which for me, as a drinker, was passed out. The only problem with that was, often, I was blacked out long before I passed out, and I had no reservations, filter, inhibitions, or clear moral compass. I could only limit and try to control my environment to limit the chance and likelihood of doing damage – to myself and/or who knows what else.

Beth told me of one particularly scary night out bar hopping with some friends. Things were going okay, until they walked to the final dance club for the night. That was the last thing that she remembers. As she explains it to me, that is when the "black curtain" closed over. The next thing she knew she was waking up, still very much intoxicated, in the drunk tank.

Although that was several months ago now, Beth has no recollection of the events that led up to her being placed in the drunk tank that night. She is very thankful that she was only held until 6 a.m., and then was released without further incident because she knows it could have been a completely different story. In fact, when she was sharing this with me, I could see her shuddering at the memory, and her physical reaction spoke volumes about what her body was remembering about that evening, even when her conscious memory couldn't remember anything.

After we spoke about this incident, and a few others which had caused her concern, Beth made a healthy choice for herself and decided that she had experienced enough with alcohol in her life. She was now going to make room for more positive experiences and new things, which would allow her to expand her horizons and meet new people – people who would share similar interests and a lifestyle outside of drinking and the bar scene. This was going to include checking out the Alcoholics Anonymous program as well. She had friends who already attended and were only too happy to pick her up for meetings. She told me after her second meeting that she felt she would continue to go, as she heard good stuff and met good people there. I'm really proud of her and happy to hear that – as I've said earlier, it works if you work it, and it's worth it because you are worth it! Beth has just been given her thirty-day sobriety medallion, and I'm so proud of her.

Anxiety in My Life

I have experienced such crippling anxiety in life during the early years of my recovery that it would literally paralyze me. I would be immobilized and not able to function. I can remember one evening, in particular, I had been walking down the sidewalk heading towards a recovery meeting I would normally attend during the day-time. During the day, I felt more comfortable with arriving late and leaving early because of the anxiety I would get when I would go out at night in the dark by myself, especially in the fall and winter when it would get dark so early. Sometimes it would be really difficult for me to overcome my anxieties and be able to show up alone. This one evening, I did manage to get into my car and make my way to the hall where the AA meetings were held, but when I pulled into the parking spot, the familiar taste of metal flooded my mouth. My temperature jumped at least twenty degrees immediately, it seemed. Next, my heart started to beat very quickly, and I could feel the pumping and pressure pounding in my head – bump, bump, bump, bump – almost faster than I could keep up with, tapping on the steering wheel as though I were playing the drums. But this was not fun music I was making. I was having a panic attack, and if I wasn't able to calm myself down soon, I may have ended up with a muscle spasm. I was in big trouble and could have potentially ended up in the hospital for intravenous muscle relaxant medication inevitably leading to terrible, wicked headaches and then the suffering would truly have begun all because I did not have the skills or capacity to consciously relax or self-soothe.

Thankfully, on that particular evening, I prayed and prayed more, and eventually, I relaxed enough to drive myself home safely after quite some time, and no one ever knew that I was sitting out in the parking lot that night. Well, no one other than my Creator! It was thanks to my connection and belief, as fragile as it was then, that I was able to get home on the wings of spirituality.

In light of these personal experiences and these two amazing and very effective therapies, I want to say this – I have made three very serious attempts at suicide and all three were thwarted by what I have come to know as my Higher Power, Creator, or God. I can't and won't understand the *why* behind why I feel it is so important that I share this with you here, but I do, so I will, and it is not to be dramatic or to seek attention. It is to emphasize that each time, the spirit ensured that I was incapable of being successful in my attempts. I now understand it was so I could continue my own work of recovery from BPD, to heal, and then to be able to develop FORDitude, write this book, and dedicate the rest of my life in service of others, helping them to heal from BPD, and start to love their lives.

Dependency in Childhood

Children don't have the skills developed to cope with emotional pain. They can handle a broken arm much better than a broken heart. They rely heavily on a defense mechanism called repression to push the emotional wound deep into their unawareness, or subconscious mind. This is called emotional woundedness.

Severe cases of emotional wounding come from emotional,

physical, and or psychological abuse and neglect. In these cases, the household becomes a dangerous place.

The neural networks of kids who grow up in abusive situations have to focus on survival. There's no real opportunity to be a normal kid.

One rule of thumb about growing up in a dysfunctional family is that it is *not* okay to ask directly for what you need or to expect to get it. And when or if you do dare to ask for what you need, you are likely to get the opposite, so you aren't likely to make that mistake again.

The brain records and keeps track of behaviors that help the child get what she needs, and they get recorded in neural networks we call survival skills. It is the magnificent ability of the brain to adapt to its environment that helps kids survive in a chaotic home.

Unfortunately, those same survival skills of "don't talk," don't trust," and "don't feel," along with hyper-vigilance and emotional dysregulation will, in later years, get in the way of healthy intimate relationships, emotions, and job performance.

Because these children don't feel safe, they can't relax and are always on alert, scanning the environment for danger. Their anxiety level is very high and "tuned in" to everything going on around them. They can't play because they can't relax, and this will interfere with their growth as playing is how children learn and grow along normal developmental lines.

Growing up, I swore that my child would never experience or be exposed to the effects that alcohol and alcoholism had on me. I managed to keep that promise to myself, for the most part, at least until the very end of my drinking when my daughter was a teenager. She only ever saw me drunk a handful of times. The damage that was caused to my precious young daughter was a result of my tragic accident and injury when she had just turned four years old. Brianna was always quite shy and was the type to hide behind my leg and needed a lot of reassurance. This was not surprising considering that her father and I separated when she was only two years old.

She didn't know how to process what happened when I got injured and our lives got completely turned upside down any more than I did – only I didn't realize it at the time. I also didn't realize that she was going to be so impacted by this event. I understood how my new reality of chronic pain impacted me, but I did not realize the massive effect it had on the instability and subsequent fears that would become a huge part of Brianna's life. She had to bear witness to her only caregiver, her mom, being incapacitated in bed for days at a time with migraines and muscle spasms that rendered her completely immobile. She became so afraid that I was not going to be okay and that I was going to be hurt further that she could not sleep. When she would, she'd often wake up in the middle of the night, in a panic attack, and walk through the whole house, looking for things that I might trip over and fall on. She would obsessively clear off the steps and remove anything from places she thought I'd trip.

I tell this difficult story as an example of the way trauma manifests in children's behaviours. In my daughter's case, the stress in her young life manifested in her obsessive actions, her only way of coping with her worries. She did everything in her power to make sure that she kept me, her safety, as safe as she possibly could. Even then, she could never truly be a "normal", unaffected kid, as she was constantly scanning her environment for perceived dangers. She continues to bravely deal with the ways our circumstances affected her development to this day, and I could not be prouder of her.

Idealization

In order to feel safe – even in an unsafe environment – very young children use a subconscious defense called idealization. In other words, little kids put their parents up on a pedestal and see them as perfect, all-knowing, and all-powerful god-like creatures. This makes them feel safe and like "nothing can get to me since I am protected by a god-like creature." In the innocent mind of a child, "god-like creatures" are perfect – they are beyond reproach. This was very much how I saw my father, and as kids, my sisters and I called him Oz, the mighty and powerful. I did not think he could do any wrong and thought of him as god-like and perfect.

I guess it boils down to this: as a child, you cannot say to yourself "well, Dad has a drinking problem – that's about him, not me. I don't have to let it cause abandonment issues when he breaks his promises and yells at me all the time." No, in the mind of a child, it goes more like this, "If I were a better kid, Dad wouldn't drink" or, "If I was a better kid, Mom wouldn't be mad at me so much" or, "Daddy, please don't leave again. I'll be good this time. I promise!"

Because of idealization, young children can make sense of abandonment issues, not the other way around – it has to be about the child. Parents have all the power, and the child has none. The child is totally submitted and committed to the parent. As a result, the child begins to develop a sense of defectiveness that grows along with the emotional wound.

So, if the original pain of abandonment is seen as an emotional wound, then shame is an emotional infection so to speak, that sets in on top of the wound – a little closer to the surface of awareness, yet still hidden beneath it.

This shame has a voice, and it grows stronger as the abandonment issues get bigger over time. The child's self-talk begins to sound like this, "No one could ever love me" or, "What's wrong with me?" or, "I'm not good enough," and the child truly feels unlovable.

Shame-Based Family Systems

The child now has a firmly established a network of shame and defectiveness that we know as the Internal Critic or negative self-talk. It contains variations of the abandonment issues such as limiting beliefs, fears of abandonment, physiology, coping skills, and memories of shame.

This network, like any other network, gets "triggered" by internal and external anchors which could be anything – a sight, sound, feeling, smell, or taste – that reminds the child of shame or defectiveness. To this day, I can still feel my father's hand on top of my head pushing down while telling me that "children are meant to be seen and not heard". I have spent my life struggling to find the right balance in using my voice. I would either talk too much or say nothing.

In a shame-based family system, these internal messages of shame are confirmed by the parents. Sometimes the confirmations are more subtle, like veiled threats of abandonment, double-bind messages, gestures that convey contempt for the child, discounting the child's feelings, and other nonverbal expressions of disdain that the child is feeling but not actually saying.

By the time the child becomes a teenager with the ability to understand that Mom and Dad are *not* the perfect god-like creatures they were once thought to be, the neural networks of abandonment issues, shame, and defectiveness are already firmly established. Couple this with the fact that teenagers are naturally experiencing a need to rebel against the family – a normal rite of passage – what you might call the "life sucks" network – it affects the teenager's whole experience of life as well as her role in it. Your emotions provide you with the "energy to move" in a certain direction. The emotions of anger, bitterness, and resentment contain a lot of energy. That energy must go somewhere, and most often it ends up going nowhere good.

The term "false-self" is used because it is just that – false, as in a *not* true, manufactured, self-rooted in abandonment issues. It only feels like who you are. It feels that way because the wound is emotional in nature. As I grew older, I would put on masks as required to fill the roles of who I had to be, and looking back, I marvel that I was able to "act as if" and be whoever I was with, who I wanted to be, or who I needed to be.

And, if you are anything like me, I was well into my 40s before I could fathom that my father was just another human being doing the best he could, and not the man on the pedestal who could do no wrong I believed him to be for so long. It's been a long, painful journey of growth and acceptance, but one that I am so grateful to have begun. I would never have dreamt we would have been able to heal our relationship to the degree that we have. I believe that most people will do their best until they know better, and then they will do better. My father and I have both worked on our personal recoveries over the years, and I feel that the level of healing that we have been able to reach is due to the fact that we have each grown so much in our own right and recoveries that we continually encourage each other in our mutual recovery and conversation to be the family who not only got sick together, but is an example of one who gets well together. My Dad is far from perfect, and with tears rolling down his cheeks he has admitted to making mistakes, but I'm most proud of the man he is today – the man who continues to stand by me and does the best he can with what he has to encourage and support me. He respects my boundaries and allows me space when I need it.

The how we do it, remains constant also. Honest in all things, period, no exceptions, and errors by omission are still errors. Openminded to all possibilities and all outcomes, as we are both aware that neither of us experienced either's reality. And willingness to consider all ways and to always be considerate.

It's not until you significantly heal your abandonment, shame, and contempt that you will be able to feel differently about yourself and then begin to heal into the person you are and were supposed to be all along. I remember always feeling so angry that I, not either of my two sisters, ended up the only one in our family with all the "issues" and thought it so unfair. It has been quite a journey of recovery from my multiple traumas, my injuries, my alcoholism, as well as my BPD. But, believe it or not, I can honestly say, today, that I wouldn't change a thing, and I am grateful for all of it – the lessons, the experiences and, most of all, the growth into the person I am today.

Acceptance Is the Answer

Beth shared with me a story of a time where she found herself the target of a smear campaign by so-called friends. People she respected and trusted had said untrue and hurtful things about her. Worst yet, they had looked at her innocently and denied they had said or done anything wrong. It happened more than once, and it hurt her deeply.

She told me that she really wanted to work through this issue and move forward in her life. It had taken enough of her time and caused her too much pain and grief as it was. We spent time discussing the concept of "Acceptance is the answer" and how so much of life is in our response to what is happening. As that is the only real ability, we have to effectively deal with it. You may have heard the old saying, "Life is 5 percent what happens and 95 percent how you respond to it." That, in my opinion, is so true! Acceptance is of the same mindset, and I'll take it one step further and say that my life has improved so much more since I learned the second part, which I shared with Beth as well. Acceptance is not approval. Read that again.

You don't have to approve or like or agree with what is happening in your life, but you can be reassured if you do not accept it – life will become much more difficult as a result of that. So, although she was devastated by these so-called friends, Beth decided that she would be much better off accepting what happened, realizing that it was not about her as much as it was entirely about those people not being worthy of her trust. She acknowledged to herself that she wasn't okay with what happened or how much it had hurt her, and then she made a conscious choice to let it go anyway. In fact, she and I have discussed that she feels so much less stress now, less animosity and is thankful to instead feel stronger and be more grounded because of the experience.

> *And acceptance is the answer to all my problems today. When I am disturbed, it is because I find some person, place, thing, or situation – some fact of my life – unacceptable to me, and I can find no serenity until I accept that person, place, thing, or situation as being exactly the way it is supposed to be at this moment. Nothing, absolutely nothing, happens in God's world by mistake. Until I could accept my alcoholism, I could not stay sober; unless I accept life completely on life's terms, I cannot be happy. I need to concentrate not so much on what needs to be changed in the world as on what needs to be changed in me and in my attitudes.*
>
> *—Alcoholics Anonymous, Basic Text*

Chapter 8

Step 5

Integrated Healing Approaches

"What I want for my fans and for the world, for anyone who feels pain, is to lean into that pain and embrace it as much as they can and begin the healing process."

Lady Gaga

Healing with Art

With over thirty years of sobriety now, my father has discovered an incredible talent for painting. Although I don't share his level of talent or sobriety – yet – I have also realized that I really enjoy allowing myself the freedom of expression that a blank canvas and paint brushes provide for me. I can create anything that my heart desires.

Several years ago, I had taken a healing through art course, and I found it to be incredibly beneficial – especially working with the little girl inside of me, who needed to be helped and healed, as well. I continued to pick up my paint brushes when the inspiration struck me, and I love that I am not held back any more by the feeling that I will never be as good as my father. That may be the case, but it's not a competition between us in my mind and that is what matters more than my level of talent. It's simply about giving myself permission to do something that I enjoy and not find an excuse to hide because of someone else.

I would really encourage you to consider looking locally for a venue that hosts a periodic "Paint Night," which are lots of fun and are a great way to express your inner most Picasso for less than fifty bucks and in just two hours. It is not about anything other than freedom to enjoy yourself and not to critique the finished result. Any medium, anything you can use your hands to shape or form, is bound to hold enjoyment for you even if it is just to relax a little as you work a ball of clay over a wheel and slowly begin to form the round shape that it will be once it is finished as a flower vase. So, whatever it is you may get your hands dirty in, have fun with it.

This reminds me of one of my favorite seasonal healing activities – gardening, plants, and flowers. Any time that I can spend with my hands in the soil and plants or moss and bark, I am literally in my element. I would also suggest that you spend as much time outside as you are able to, and if at all possible, try some gardening activities. What is your favorite perennial? Annual? House plant? I think one of the reasons that I love my plants as much as I do is because I like to talk to the plants. I will blame that on living alone, and we will leave it at that!

Expressive Journaling: Unlocking the Power of Gratitude

Gratitude is gold. Often, the lessons we learn are from people with big hearts and we never know who our next teacher will be. When I was living in Annapolis Valley, Nova Scotia, from the age of five to twelve, I walked to the school bus every morning, and, on the way, I stopped and collected my friend and neighbor, Shirley. Shirley had far from an easy life, and I took her under my wing and sort of thought of myself as her protector. She had suffered from Scarlett Fever when she was a baby and as a result, was noticeably crippled on her left side. Shirley had a great attitude and a heart of gold, but not everyone saw her as I did. Not everyone took the time to get to know her, or, was willing to look beyond her circumstances. Sadly, some of the kids at our school would be quite cruel and say unkind things to her. She lit up my days, and no matter how awful things were at my home, she always made me feel better. I knew that things could always been worse.

Some of my best and happiest memories, to this day, are spending time in the elementary school yard with Wanda and Shirley, my longest and best friends. I am so grateful for the bond and connection that I formed with these two incredible women, both very different from very different worlds than mine, but we were three amigos that were always there for each other – no matter what! We had each other's backs, and at that point in my life, everyone thought my life was so great, and I could not tell them otherwise – I knew better. But I also knew I had a safe place with my two friends, and they would always accept me and be there for me. We would sing our hearts out while swinging as high as we could. We would make each other laugh and smile and encourage one another, and, somehow, after spending time in their company, it always made going home more bearable. I didn't know at the time that what I was feeling was gratitude. I didn't have a name for it, but I knew how it felt. It was when we would start laughing that I would feel my heart swell. I'd be feeling wonderful and feeling joy. I'd come to know and learn that gratitude will make you healthier and happier. Furthermore, if you make repeated gestures of gratitude, daily, they will accumulate into a sense of well-being and happiness.

Every day, gratitude in action can be a fun exercise and the benefits and payoffs are happiness all around. You can start with:

- Starting a gratitude journal and listing three things you're grateful for each day
- Giving a thank you note to someone who is not expecting it
- Giving a bouquet of fall flowers to someone you appreciate
- Setting a grateful example and saying "thank you" to your kids for helping with table-setting or toy cleanup
- Lighting a candle and focusing on a recent blessing
- Bringing dinner to someone who nurtures others (e.g. Soup and bread are perfect for sharing)
- Making collages of the people, places, and opportunities for which you're most grateful and laminating your creations to use as a placemat
- Taking a walk through the woods and being thankful for the changing seasons
- Going online to merchants who make or sell objects you love and leaving a positive review (the merchant and the next shopper will appreciate it)
- Planning a date night with your spouse or child and tuning in to what makes them happy

In order to be happy with yourself, you have to truly make peace and love yourself. We often put the key to our happiness and contentment in someone else's pocket and it's time to reach back in there and reclaim what belongs to you.

I can't possibly count the number of journals (double digits) that I have written in over the years. I have written letters to God, letters to my younger self, letters to my dad, letters to the men I was in relationships with, and to whoever else I needed to communicate with that I didn't feel capable of having a conversation with – for whatever reason. I knew that by writing my thoughts on paper it was a safe place, for me, to start and maybe even finish the communication. There are specific exercises that you can do when working on different parts of your trauma or healing, and they have been proven to be very effective. It is always up to the composer whether or not the material will be shared afterward or destroyed.

"Gratitude" is a poem and a lovely example of art in recovery, and healing in art, written by a very dear long-time family friend, Elva. She is a beautiful soul who has inspired me over the many years I have known her. She has been in recovery for several years now and has written many healing, thoughtful, and inspiring poems during her sobriety, showing her gratitude for the fellowship of AA and the friends she has made along the way. I am so blessed to be counted among them and even more so that she has shared her words, of which I totally agree, and her gift of gratitude with us here. Many thanks and much love to you Elva xox!

Gratitude

Forever grateful I shall be
For what AA has given me,
It gave me life, it gave me hope
It also taught me how to cope
It brought me from the gates of hell
To this place where I now dwell,
Among people of my own kind
The most loving friends I could ever find.
So full of hate and guilt I came
So full of remorse and full of shame,
You didn't tell me to go away
You welcomed me in and asked me to stay.
You showed me love and led the way
You gave me hope for another day,
You asked for nothing more from me
You just showed me the way to sobriety.
A higher power I also have found
Whose love for me has no bounds,
His will I try to do every day
For the steps have told me, this is the way.
Although I slip sometimes in my mind
Through you and AA the answers I find,
Because of the love you give to me
I pray this is where I will always be.
The longer I'm here the more I'm aware
How much you and God have showed me you care,
So thank you dear friends for showing me the way,
I know with your help I'll be here to stay
As long as I work at it day after day.

Music

I don't know where I'd be without music in my life – it can soothe the soul, bring me such comfort, or it can pump me up when I need a boost of energy to help me get going. I use music on my way to work in my car to bring me up on the way in and to help me decompress on the way home at the end of a busy day. It is always there, and with just a word or a hint of a melody, can transport me back in time to a place, or a space, pleasant and nice or sad and lonely. So, choosing what to listen to, as in all things, is important. I personally love to sing and dance, and both have helped me tremendously in my journey of healing. I would encourage you to be daring and bold and be willing to have fun and be heard – express yourself and shake your booty!

Just ask any of my family or friends, and anyone of them will tell you that my favorite thing to do anytime, anywhere is *karaoke* – oh yeah! For me, there is no better enjoyment, no game I want to play more, and it's a great release of my pent-up energy. I let it all out through the microphone for a few moments – I sing like I'm living my absolute best life ever because in those few minutes, the world is my stage and I am loving it! It doesn't matter if you are a great singer or not – not everyone was born with pipes like Carrie Underwood, Pink, or Gwen Stephani, and you know what? That's okay! It is only about enjoying your time with the microphone and not caring or worrying about what anyone thinks about what you sound like – what matters is how it makes you feel. Those people will forget it in five minutes, but you won't, and that's the magic!

Visualize

Visualization is a powerful tool that you can use anytime to help you when you are having a tough moment or stuck in a bad spot. I use an exercise that helps me a lot, no matter the circumstances, and it is to simply close my eyes and picture myself enjoying being in one of my most favorite places, sitting in Sean's peddle boat on Trout Lake back home in Nova Scotia, where I was born. I still can hear the water hitting the sides of boat and feel the bits of water splashing up on me while I can see the sun reflecting off the magnificent blue water. I can smell the campfires burning and can almost taste hot dogs and the marshmallows roasting. The more details you bring in, the more real it will feel. If you consider using your five senses – how it looks, how it feels, what sounds are there, the tastes associated with it – it allows you to ground yourself and more easily move through difficult and painful emotions and sensations.

Imagery

As I learned from *Surviving Trauma*, Bellaruth writes that "guided imagery is a deliberate daydreaming designed to evoke rich, multi-sensory fantasy and memory in order to create a deeply immersive, receptive mind-state ideal for catalyzing desired changes in the mind, body, psyche, and spirit." It is gentle, but very powerful and can yield instant results. It has been found to reduce anxiety and depression, lower blood pressure, reduce cholesterol, speed up healing from cuts, fractures, and burns, beef up immune function, reduce pain from arthritis and fibromyalgia, and many other medical conditions and situations. It even has a positive effect with improving eating disorders, infertility, weight loss, and concentration in developmentally disabled adults.

It is effective in part as it can sidestep linear thinking and logical assumptions and jostle defeating self-concepts while floating soft appealing reminders of health, strength, meaning, and hope. The imagery is taken mostly by the right hemisphere of the brain, the emotion-based channels, using your capacity for sensing, perceiving, feeling and apprehending, rather than your left brain that handles thinking, judging, analyzing, and deciding.

I use imagery regularly and often on a daily basis. So much so, it is happening without me even realizing it now. I find it so helpful and effective in soothing myself in times of heightened feelings and emotions. Before, I would have just continued to spin out of control with no healthy outlet or coping skills, and it would have gotten progressively worse and taken me much longer to resolve my feelings and return to any sense of wellness or semblance of calm.

I had an early start with this from my days as a competitive figure skater. My coach would talk to me about practicing my skating routines and jumps in my mind. Little I realized what it was she was actually having me do, and it certainly did help improve my technique on the ice.

Most recently, the best example I can use to illustrate the effectiveness of this is Bianca Andreescu, the nineteen-year-old Canadian who upset the tennis world earlier this year when she surprised everyone, not the least of which was Serena Williams, when she won a Grand Slam singles title by beating the greatest female tennis player of all time. Bianca is quoted in one of her interviews after her stunning victory saying that her mother had taught her the value and power of imagery. She believes in it so much that over the years, she has written herself checks of increasing value to support her belief, faith in herself, and her talent and ability – she certainly proved that it paid off handsomely having won over six million dollars. I share that as just one more example of how this type of work can be so beneficial in our lives.

The Benefits of Exercise

Exercise can work as effectively as an antidepressant medication to treat depression, but without the side effects. Much research shows the benefits of exercise compared to medication for people with depression. A daily fifteen to thirty-minute moderate exercise to get your blood pumping and your heart rate up will get your endorphins flowing. It's a natural way to use your body's chemicals to your advantage. Any type of activity, from a brisk walk, jog, or a run, to any type of sports team or solo sport that gets you out and involved is a great way to accomplish this goal.

According to www.helpguide.org, exercise can improve not just your physical health, physique, improve your waist-line, sex life, and add years to your life, but it can also enormously improve your sense of well-being. Those of us who exercise regularly tend to feel more energetic throughout the day, sleep better at night, have better memories, and feel more relaxed and positive about ourselves and our lives. Regular exercise is a powerful medicine, which can have a profoundly positive impact on depression, anxiety, and many other mental health issues.

Studies at Harvard TH Chan School of Public Health have found that running for fifteen minutes a day or walking for an hour reduces the risk of major depression by 26 percent and relieves depression symptoms. Research also shows that maintaining an exercise schedule can prevent you from relapsing. There are many reasons why exercise is a powerful depression fighter, most importantly, it promotes all kinds of changes in the brain, including neural growth, reduced inflammation, and new activity patterns that promote feelings of calm and well-being. It releases endorphins, powerful chemicals in your brain that energize your spirit and make you feel good. Exercise can also serve as a distraction and can allow you to find some quiet time to break out of the cycle of negative thoughts that feed depression. It is an effective tool for natural and effective anti-anxiety treatment as it relieves tension and stress.

While exercising you will notice all sensations, like your feet hitting the ground or the rhythm of your breathing or the wind on your skin, for instance, by adding the element of mindfulness to your exercise. By allowing yourself to really focus on you and how it feels as you exercise, you'll not only improve your physical condition, but you'll also be able to interrupt the constant flow of worries running through your head. The same endorphins that make you feel better also help you concentrate, feel mentally sharp, and stimulate the growth of new brain cells.

Regular activity is an investment in your mind, body, and soul, and when it becomes habit it can foster your sense of self-worth and make you feel strong and powerful. You'll feel better about your appearance, and as you meet your goals, you'll feel a sense of achievement and accomplishment. Even short burst of exercise anytime in the day can help you regulate your sleep patterns, but if you exercise at night, relaxing exercises such as yoga or gentle stretching can help promote sleep. When faced with a mental or emotional challenge in your life exercise can help you cope in a healthy way instead of resorting to alcohol, drugs, or other negative behaviors that ultimately will only make your symptoms worse.

Spend time in nature swimming, bird watching, combing the beach look for shells or collecting rocks are all great ways to spend part of your day. Yoga, qigong, tai chi, or any other martial art is a great way to combine mindfulness, breathing work, and exercise in one activity. Body work, as required, such as massage, reiki, pressure points, craniosacral therapy, or whatever modality suits your individual needs can also be beneficial.

If it means doing a little something or nothing, always air on the side of a little something is better than nothing and build from there. Remember, you eat an elephant one bite at a time. It's the little victories that will add up and allow you to accomplish bigger ones, but it always starts with the first step.

Sleep Hygiene

Having suffered from sleep issues myself, I know how difficult they can be to deal with. In my case, it was more often a case of needing a lot of sleep versus suffering from insomnia. Recently, however, I dealt with a period of insomnia that lasted over two months, and it was horrendous; the effects were far reaching. I truly had no idea how awful and impactful not sleeping would be on my body, mind, and spirit day-to-day. I have a much greater understanding and incredible empathy for anyone who experiences the effects of sleep disturbances regularly.

I had done much research on this subject, previously, through a course I took on natural medicine and natural healing and more recently, during my own bout of insomnia. The information remains the same, and the good news is that you can set up a good sleep management system without the use of medication – excuse the pun, but it won't happen overnight!

The Role and Function of Sleep

Sleep is essential just like air, water, and food. When necessary, people can cope without sleep for periods of time, but research shows that it is important for general physical health, restoring energy, repairing injuries or illness, growth, psychological well-being and mood, concentration, memory, work performance, and getting along well with others and in life. The average person will do well with seven and half to eight hours of sleep per night, while others function well with only four to five hours.

Your Sleep Routine

Sleep hygiene describes good sleep habits and strategies designed to enhance sleeping and provide long-term solutions to sleep difficulties. These tips will assist you in developing a good routine to establish sleep habits:

- Be consistent and sleep when you are sleepy
- Get up, instead of lying there wide awake, and try to go down for sleep again later
- Avoid stimulants like caffeine and nicotine four to six hours before bed
- Avoid alcohol four to six hours before bed
- Use your bed for sleeping only
- Don't take naps through the day
- Have a wind down ritual, such as taking a hot bath before bed
- No clock watching
- Use a sleep diary to track your sleep

All these great tips are useful but will require putting some thought into setting yourself up for success and winding down properly for the evening. A period of brisk activity or exercise is recommended earlier in the day/evening, followed by setting up a schedule, such as taking a soothing bath with essential oils, having a cup of tea, doing nighttime meditation, and not using any electronics (including television). A consistent routine is always best when possible. Your brain likes routine and does its best work when it knows what to expect.

Importance of Breath Work

On average, we take 23,000 breaths a day. We do this action more than *anything* else we do, and yet, it is something very few of us practice. It has been proven that conscious breathing and practicing breath work throughout the day is extremely beneficial.

"Feelings come and go like clouds in a windy sky.
Conscious breathing is my anchor."
— Thich Nhat Hanh

Focus on your breathing when you are upset or stressed. Your breathing becomes quick and shallow, which, in turn, causes other reactions in your body. Some of these reactions are referred to as the fight or flight syndrome. Breathing deeply and slowly instantly calms you down mentally as well as physically.

Breathing infuses you with life force energy and opens your chakras, portals, and your hearts. Working with your breath is so easy, but few actually believe in its effectiveness and strength.

The basic breath exercise I'd like to share and teach you is to simply take a full deep breath in through one nostril (right) while covering the other, exhale out through your mouth, and then release. Change and breathe through the other nostril (left), and then hold the other side closed, then exhale through your mouth and repeat that exercise series for five full sessions (for each side).

"Being aware of your breath forces you into the pres-
ent moment — the key to all inner transformation.
Whenever you are conscious of the breath, you are
absolutely present. You may notice that you cannot
think and be aware of your breathing. Conscious
breathing stops your mind."
— Eckhart Tolle

Next, do a square breathing exercise, which is to simply breathe in through your nose for a count of four and hold and pause for the same count of four. Inhale for a count of four, hold for a count of four, exhale for a count of four, hold for a count of four, inhale for a count of four, and exhale for a count of four. Or, in other words, inhale two-three-four, hold two-three-four, exhale two-three-four, hold two-three-four, inhale two-three-four, hold two-three-four, and exhale two-three-four.

A Lesson in Framing

The longer I live, the more I realize the impact of attitude on life. Attitude, to me, is more important than facts. It is more important than the past, than education, than money, than circumstances, than failures, than successes, than what other people think or say or do. It is more important than appearance, giftedness, or skill. It will make or break a company...a church...a home. The remarkable thing is, we have a choice every day regarding the attitude we will embrace for that day. We cannot change our past...we cannot change the fact that people will act in a certain way. We cannot change the inevitable. The only thing we can do is play on the one string we have, and that is our attitude...I am convinced that life is 10% what happens to me and 90% how I react to it, and so it is with you...we are in charge of our attitudes.

– Unknown

When I was still living in Nova Scotia, I had been terminated from my position as account manager/technical recruiter for a large national IT staffing company. I wasn't let go because of my performance, quite the opposite, in fact. I was earning accolades and quarterly bonuses equivalent to an average professional salary with my snazzy office in one of the most prestigious waterfront penthouse offices in downtown Halifax, Nova Scotia. I was returning home one day from an appointment at a pain clinic that I had attended with my husband, Ken, only to find a registered letter in my mailbox advising me that I was no longer employed. It did not provide a specific reason, but it said that I was not meeting the requirement of being in the office. I did not have any sick time benefits and because I was the only person looking after the entire Atlantic region for information technology specialists and contract staffing, both as an account manager and as a technical recruiter for Nova Scotia, New Brunswick, and Prince Edward Island, this meant that while I could not be terminated because of my illness, when I wasn't there, no work was getting done. So, they gave me a severance package and off I went – broken open even further now. It is truly only right that as I write these words, I am realizing that it was from that brokenness that things went from bad to much, much worse. But through this experience I learned a lesson in framing.

Framing is so much more about how you respond to what is happening to you than it is about what is happening in the world around you. For example, let's look at how this happens in the small variation of the words a doctor could use to describe your chances of success during a surgery. In one situation, the doctor could say, "95 percent of patients who have this surgery recover fine and live," while in another situation, the same doctor could tell another person that, "5 percent of patients who have this surgery die." Although the statistics are the same, the patients' perceptions are very different as those who heard the 5 percent risk of dying perceived their risk to be much greater. This is a valuable lesson that we can use to help our conscious mind interpret information by framing things as positively as possible with just a slight change in wording while maintaining the fact.

What You Focus on Enlarges

You've probably heard the age-old question about the grass being greener on the other side of the fence, but the question is why is that? I like to believe that it is because that grass is being tended to, fertilized, aerated, watered, and generally cared for and, therefore, it is healthier and will grow better. Essentially, whatever we focus on and give our full attention to gets bigger and better, hence why the grass is greener. That is also the very basic concept of mindfulness, which we will explore further in more detail later.

Letting Go

In order to move forward, you must become willing to let go of all that is holding you back. It is not easy to know what it means to let go or what you need to let go of. The following is a list I have had for many years that I was gifted in my early recovery from my addiction to alcohol. I do not know the author to give proper credit; however, as is with most of the recovery literature, it is free for the taking and sharing. So, in that spirit, I will share it here unaltered:

- To let go does not mean to stop caring, it means I can't do it for someone else.
- To let go is not to cut myself off, it's the realization that I can't control another.
- To let go is not to enable, but to allow learning from natural consequences.
- To let go is to admit powerlessness, which means the outcome is not in my hands.
- To let go is not to try to change or blame one another, it's to make the most of myself.
- To let go is not to care for, but to care about.
- To let go is not to fix, bot to be supportive.
- To let go is not to judge, but to allow another to be a human being.
- To let go is not to be in the middle and arrange all the outcomes, but to allow others to affect their destinies.
- To let go is not to be protective, it's to permit another to face reality.
- To let go is not to deny, but to accept.
- To let go is not to nag, scold or argue, but instead to search out my own shortcomings and correct them.
- To let go is not to adjust everything to my own desires, but to take each day as it comes and cherish myself in it.
- To let go is not to criticize or regulate anybody, but to try to become what I dream I can be.
- To let go is not to regret the past, but to grow and live for the future.

· To let go is to fear less and love more.

Judgement

Why do we as people feel the need to judge other people based on nothing more than ignorance or supposition? We make assumptions based largely on opinions and appearances when we have no idea what is going on for that person on the inside. We are completely unaware of what is going on inside that person's body, head, house, relationships, feelings, or world, of which we are far more likely to do more harm than any good.

Why, as a society, are we not so quick to embrace the idea or concept of "assume best intentions" until you have proof of the contrary? It would be such a kinder, caring and much nicer place and space to be in, and I believe that it would have a direct impact on the number of people who decide to withdraw from society. When in doubt, ask the questions to confirm instead of drawing conclusions that may or may not be correct. Communication is a two-way street, and, like driving, we all have a responsibility to ensure that we are doing our part, properly and safely.

I have often thought, as has been my own situation with an invisible disability, that most days I can look okay from the outside but be totally falling apart on the inside, and no one would have a clue. That is so long as I don't talk and then begin to cry because, if so, then all bets are off. That's the giveaway for me, and it becomes evident, quickly, that there's a lot going on under the facade.

I like to use the analogy of walking into the forest and walking around in amazement and wonder just appreciating the woods for what they are – a mixture of all different kinds of trees, shrubs, bushes, and plants. Some are tall, big, short, bent, broken, dark in color, evergreen, big leaves, no leaves, falling over, standing straight, partially rotten, bearing fruit, housing nests, and the list could go on and on. But when have you ever heard anyone walking in the beautiful forest exclaim about the differences in the trees? I would suggest to you, not once have you ever heard anyone doing that. Not once has anyone ever thought to judge the trees in the forest against each other – we simply appreciate each one for its individual beauty and uniqueness and for what its purpose is. What does each tree or shrub offer to the forest? What does it bring to the environment around it? Does it make good ground cover for rabbits to hide from their natural predators? Does the tree offer a great place for majestic eagles to build nests and hatch their young? Why is it that we as a society are so quick to jump to criticize and judge others without knowing the struggles and strife that brought each of us to where we are today? Instead, we are more seemingly interested in making ourselves feel better at someone else's expense. I really hope that we can start paying attention to what we are thinking and doing to not judge ourselves too harshly going forward, but also to assume the best for others, as well, and bear in mind, that we can effect more positive change in the world by being kind and doing good.

And even going further, let's imagine experiencing this beautiful forest with all of our senses. Begin by imagining the feeling of the rough sensation of the prickly, evergreen needles in your hands, the smell of the dank and musky moss that covers the bark on the base of the trees. See the magnificent eagles soaring overhead with their wings spread wide as they glide effortlessly. Hear the sound of the bubbling brook as the water rushes downwards over the rocks and pebbles before it flows out to the wide mouth of the lake. And finally, taste the salt on your lips from the sweat that has been collecting as you've been walking strenuously uphill to the amazing hilltop where you are now perched and enjoying this amazing forest scene.

So, let's start with small steps, and you will be amazed by what you notice in yourself and how quickly it offers you back a feeling of warmth and kindness. This is a golden oldie – never do to others what you would not wish to have done to you. Be like an oak and stand tall and proud of who you are and what you are capable of doing.

Different Lenses

A very important insight I gleaned years ago that has been so helpful to me was realizing that we each see the world through our very own set of lenses. Each of us have arrived where we are today, bringing with us the sum total of all of our experiences, relationships, family relations, education, work history, friendships, hardships, therapies, treatments, traumas, injuries, addictions, disorders, diseases, disappointments, and really, the list could go on forever, but I think you get my point. No two life experiences are identical; therefore, it would stand to reason that no two sets of life lenses could be identical either.

Listen to Your Gut Feelings

One of the most memorable events in my life by far, took place when my family and I woke up on our first day in Jerusalem when my dad got stationed there for a year. As you may know, the city of Jerusalem is built on a hill and the views are incredible. My two older sisters were still tired, dealing with jetlag, and had decided to stay in the hotel room and nap. My mom and I, however, decided to go and do some sightseeing, as Dad was already off to report in to his office at the UN Headquarters.

The very first thing we came across was a camel done up in all its finery and a handsome young man who was all too eager for us to pay him some money to let us sit on the camel so we could have our picture taken on this decked out camel.

Although, initially, I felt uncertain about the man with the camel, I thought to myself, "Don't be silly, he's here in front of the hotel. What could possibly go wrong?" And, of course, I desperately wanted to have my picture taken with the camel, but there was no way I was able to convince my mom to get on with me – no way! Not surprisingly, Mom wasn't the type to ride horses, she was afraid of heights, and this camel was at least about six and half or seven feet from the ground up.

So, we paid him the amount of money the man was asking for to allow me to sit up on the camel, and then Mom was going to take my picture. Then she was going to stand in front of the camel with me and an older gentleman that was also there was going to take our picture together, and then we'd be done. It would have been a great experience had it been that – but it wasn't!

134

As soon as Mom stepped away from the camel after we had the picture taken, the young guy who owned the camel, who I believe was in his late 20s or early 30s, very quickly launched himself up onto the camel behind me and spurred the camel on. It began trotting down the hill and away from my mom. Startled, I tried to turn around and yell at Mom to follow us, but I could not see her. The road was not only downhill, but it was on a constant turn to the right, and I couldn't even see Mom anymore. By then, I could feel his arms begin squeezing around my rib, holding me, and I know he wasn't going to let me go.

He started asking me how old I am and if I would like to live in Israel with him. At first I thought he was joking, and then I realized he wasn't. I asked him to take me back to my mom and told him that she would be worried about me and for him to please turn around now. By this point, he was now telling me that he has been waiting to find a beautiful, young, Canadian girl, like me, and he has many camels to offer my parents for me, but first he wanted to spend time alone with me. I was then on the verge of totally freaking out, realizing that I may be getting abducted, but, at this same time, I couldn't believe it was happening.

The camel's pace had picked up and it was now moving much faster, and I didn't know if I could jump off with his arms wrapped around me so tightly around me. The roads were so narrow and not weren't many people around, so I really didn't know what to do. Then all of a sudden, I can hear someone yelling, *"Stop! Stop! Stop that camel!"* and the pounding hooves of a donkey came up beside me on the camel. There was my mom holding on for her life to a dear old man, on the back of his donkey, hollering at the guy driving the camel I was on. She was yelling *"Stop that camel right now and let my daughter off immediately!"* At which time the man riding the donkey followed it up with something in his native tongue. The camel quickly stopped.

I got off as quickly as I possibly could, although it seemed to take forever for the camel to lower enough for me to jump to the ground to safety. I was never so happy and proud of my mom in my whole life, and we began the long, very tiring walk back up the hill to our hotel room.

I was exhausted, mentally, emotionally and physically after that terrifying ordeal, and I think it was one of my earliest lessons about not paying attention to my gut and "talking myself through it" because I wanted to do something so badly. I was so impatient, that I could have been harmed again because I, yet again, talked myself out of my instinct for survival.

Thank goodness that I was not violated, but it could have turned out much differently if my mom hadn't put on her superhero cape and jumped on a donkey to come and save my butt, literally. I wanted to share this story to show you the importance of listening to your gut and what it is telling you and why talking yourself through something is not a good idea.

Chapter 9

Step 6

Therapeutic Approaches

"The definition of insanity is doing the same thing over and over again and expecting a different result."

Albert Einstein

Starts with Awareness

When I was a year sober, I went to my doctor and begged for help. I was losing my mind and didn't realize that without the ability to numb my pain and feelings with alcohol, as I had been doing my whole life, I was stark raving "sober, crazy, and suicidal". As she knew of my dysfunctional childhood and the whiplash injury I had sustained in 1997, from which I was still suffering chronic pain and debilitating headaches, she recommended that I begin seeing a psychologist who specialized in treating patients with chronic pain issues and do psychotherapy. I agreed immediately, knowing I would do anything to deal with the mess in my mind and could only hope to find my solution there. The truth was, I really had no idea what was wrong with me.

It was at that time that I finally got the diagnosis of BPD that would allow my healing to begin. I finally understood why I had always felt like I had, and I had hope for the first time that I could change my behaviours and, as a result, my personality. I had hope of no longer having the disorder, which meant that I would not have to feel or act like I had anymore. Can you say *rejoice* and *relief*? Well, I probably didn't right away, but I certainly did soon after. And as I sit here now writing this, they are the two words that come to mind to best describe what I would come to know. But initially, I have to confess, my diagnosis was scary.

Stop Sign

When I began seeing Larry, my psychologist, the first thing he brought to my attention was the fact that my internal dialogue to and with myself was, quite frankly, terrible. I was not nice to myself at all. I would talk down to myself, name call, demean, minimize, etc., whether I was telling him a story from a long time ago or from a recent situation. Even if I was telling him about thoughts I was having, they always included this awful negative self-bashing. I remember that a default saying of mine was, "I don't know, I just don't f****ing know anything". I would refer to myself as a dummy or say that I was stupid and literally did not have one nice thing to think or say about myself.

The first thing he had me work on was becoming aware of the instances of this self-bashing. When I would – the goal was to visualize a stop sign and, literally, just stop the thought gently and not be further critical of myself by beating myself up or being nasty to myself for not being nice, which, of course, was my tendency to do. I bet you can relate to that one, right? Yup, that was me.

So, that's where we started with the stop sign, and from there, we moved to stop sign with a stopping thought to a changing thought to a new positive thought about myself. It wasn't particularly difficult, but it was a little tricky to first become aware and then begin to start changing the thinking pattern. With ongoing practice, in time, it will become easier, and, eventually, it will become your new vocabulary.

The Unknown Known

I realize now how little I thought of myself at that time, but I guess it isn't really surprising now that I more fully understand BPD. When there is no sense of self, it is virtually impossible to have positive self-esteem. I would marvel at the things I would realize only after Larry would help me to uncover/discover them through the many, many (did I mention the many?) hours of talk therapy. I sat in his office talking about my life, my confused thinking, and how it was incredible for me when he would inevitably be able to help me piece things together and the light bulb would turn on. But, yet, it was as though, somehow, I already knew – it just wasn't clear to me. He explained that to me, as well, as "the unknown, known." I still hear his voice in my head, and I am so incredibly grateful for the time, teaching, and tolerance he showed me during the years I was his patient.

You Are *Not* Your Thoughts

Larry also taught me that I was not my thoughts and that although I was/am in charge of my thoughts, there is a huge difference. That lesson was a big one for me at that point in my life but was a necessary step in learning to manage my mind, feelings, emotions, and ultimately my life, as I am able to do so successfully today. I am forever changed for the better for all of it, and I would not have experienced the growth and knowledge about me that I have today if it were not for him, so for that, I am truly grateful. Thank you, Larry.

Distancing Yourself from Your Thoughts

To distance yourself from your thoughts, you need to realize that your thoughts are just thoughts, and you don't have to react to them. For example, you might think, "Well, this could be the day the plane crashes." Instead of reacting to that thought, think, "that's an interesting thought", and then let that thought float away. Don't react to thoughts like that, just realize that they are only thoughts. Keep letting them float by until your anxiety subsides. Whether or not the plane crashes, worrying about it doesn't affect the outcome.

No matter how you begin managing your mind and putting worry to work for you, knowledge is power!

The first step is to know your unruly mind can be tamed. You can learn to control your racing thoughts and develop healthy habits for dealing with unpleasant emotions and events by writing your thoughts down at the beginning and end of the day to get them out of your head and on paper. You don't have to address them right then, but now you have a record of them, and you don't need to keep turning them over in your head.

Then, talk to someone who can help you solve the problem or evaluate your concern. Set aside a "thinking time" each day when you will deal with your thoughts. Practice radical acceptance. Sometimes things just are. Adopt an "It is what it is. Now, how can I improve the next moment" attitude. Quiet the internal critic and be more realistic. What is the likelihood that the sky is falling? Exercise to pull energy from your mind down to those bigger muscles.

Next, know your direction. It is easier to identify thoughts and concerns that are not worth your time and can be let go of if you know where you are headed and what is important. Examine the practicality of the thought. Is this worry or thought helping me? If so, okay, do something about it. If not, then it is impractical to get all twisted up about it.

I woke up to a minister on TV this morning who spent the entire thirty minutes telling people to send him money and God would bless them for it. Uhhh...God doesn't work that way. Did it irritate me? Yes, for a minute, but that anger was not practical. My feelings about the situation were not going to change anything. All I could do was pray that people could see the truth, and then let it go. I had other things that were demanding my energy.

Push the thoughts away (if you determine they are unhelpful). Sometimes you may have thoughts that you are going to fail, or something is going to go wrong, or you perseverate on things that didn't go right. Do your best, get your ducks in a row, and then push those thoughts away. Continuing to worry is not going to do any good. Practice effective time management so you do not feel pulled in ten different directions and stressed that you will not be able to live up to your obligations. And focus on the positive. Even though one thing may be going poorly, you likely have four or five other things that are important to you and are going well.

Remember *all* of the things you are committed to, not just the ones that are going poorly. Identify what parts of the situation you have control over (even if it's just your reaction to the situation), and view dealing with it as a challenge instead of a struggle.

Practice mindfulness identifying three things you see, three things you hear, three things you smell, and three things you feel. When you are focused on trying to identify these things, your mind cannot be thinking about other stuff. You are compelling it to change directions.

Stop assigning meaning to things and taking them personally or believing in superstitions such as, "well, because I overslept, the rest of the day is going to be a disaster too". Remember, we choose our beliefs. Pray and give control of the things that you are unable to control to your higher power or good orderly direction.

Practice Is Important

If at first you don't succeed, don't give up – get up and do it again, and again and again and again and again. This is called practice.

I began ice skating at the age of three. My two older sisters were in figure skating, so it made sense for my mom to put me in skating as well. I fell in love with it. I had a real daredevil attitude and wasn't afraid to try anything on the ice. By the age of nine, I was competing in solo events as well as precision line skating competitions. I tell you this to emphasize the importance of learning anything new and being prepared to put in the time and effort through practicing to gain the skills and experience to get good at it.

While a lot of my friends were home snuggled in their warm beds still sleeping soundly, I was already up and at the cold rink skating, practicing for at least ninety minutes two mornings a week before school, and then another two practices after school, and then more time on the weekend. This included my private lesson with my pro. I did this all at the age of ten. I knew that I would inevitably be full of bruises and bumps by the time I got off the ice, but I also knew that I would be better for it. I was progressing quickly for my age and my coach, Katrina, was impressed with my natural skills and "can do" attitude. She often asked me to demonstrate for the group because she knew I essentially had no fear, and she could tell me how to do it, and I would go out and try it. The end result didn't matter – the willingness to do it was always there, and I knew, in time, the technique would follow.

Practice, Practice, and more Practice

So, for many years and many early mornings and long hours in the cold rink, I practiced individually and with our precision line. Our hard work paid off when our team won the Nova Scotia Provincial Championships, and we were invited to Ontario to compete in the Canadians and Internationals for Precision Line Team. It was an amazing experience, and although we skated our hearts out, we were skating out of our league and came home with great memories, but no trophies.

The lessons I learned in the rink while practicing my skating, whether doing the dreaded figures or compulsory dance or my favorite freestyle, is that there is value in every minute of it. It set the stage for me to realize how important it is to put the necessary time and effort into building the foundation of whatever it is that I am building. Without it, I will not have the strength to grow the rest on top of it, and there aren't any fast tracks to anything worth having in this life. Therefore, I wake each morning and dedicate the first thirty minutes to the practice of mindfulness meditation. This prepares me for the day ahead in a calm and reflective state of mind.

What is DBT?

Dialectical behavior therapy, or DBT, was developed over thirty years ago by Dr. Marsha Linehan, PhD, as a labour of love, specifically for those patients dealing with suicide ideation (thinking) and behaviours. It has since been adopted and adapted effectively for people diagnosed with borderline personality disorder, BPD.

BPD is a severe and complex disorder characterized by pervasive instability in emotions, behavior, relationships, and thoughts. Among people who have BPD, DBT has been found to be effective in reducing suicide attempts, self-harming behaviour, suicidal ideation, psychiatric hospital admittances, feelings of hopelessness, and periods of intense anger while also increasing success of therapy working long-term, social adjustments, and overall functions in general.

Suicidal and self-harming behaviours are often exhibited to reduce painful emotions, but difficulty controlling intense emotions may lead to impulsive behaviours and unstable relationships. DBT works by helping individuals with BPD learn effective strategies for regulating emotions in order to achieve more balanced emotions, behaviors, and thoughts. DBT views BPD as a disorder of pervasive emotional dysregulation, which means the individual has frequent, intense emotional responses that are difficult to change. DBT has also been shown to effectively treat cooccurring substance use disorders, such as major depressive disorder, PTSD, bulimia, binge-eating, bipolar disorder, post-traumatic-stress disorder, and substance abuse. Of note, several recent studies have also found DBT to be effective in reducing suicidal and self-harming behaviours, suicidal ideation, and depression among adolescents exhibiting BPD traits, suggesting it may be helpful in preventing at-risk individuals from progressing and meeting full diagnostic criteria for BPD.

How DBT works

DBT is a cognitive-behavioral treatment most effective for those diagnosed with BPD and who often experience extremely intense negative emotions that are difficult to manage. These intense and seemingly uncontrollable negative emotions are often experienced when the individual is interacting with others – friends, romantic partners, or family members. People with borderline often experience a great deal of conflict in their relationships.

As its name suggests, DBT is influenced by the philosophical perspective of dialectics, which means the balancing of opposites. The therapist consistently works with the individual to find ways to hold two seemingly opposite perspectives at once, promoting balance and avoiding the all-or-nothing style of thinking. Black or white thinking instead moves to a grey area or middle of the road. In service of this balance, DBT promotes a both-and rather than an either-or outlook. The dialectic at the heart of DBT is acceptance and change.

Fundamentals of DBT

DBT is support oriented and designed to help a person identify their strengths and build on them so that the person can feel better about his or herself and her life.

DBT is cognitive based and helps individuals identify thoughts, beliefs, and assumptions that make life harder. For example, identifying thoughts and beliefs like "I have to be perfect at everything" or "If I get angry, I'm a terrible person" helps people to learn different ways of thinking that will make life more bearable so they can have thoughts like "I don't need to be perfect at things for people to care about me" or "Everyone gets angry, it's a normal emotion."

DBT is collaborative and requires constant attention to relationships between clients and staff. In DBT people are encouraged to work out problems in their relationships with their therapist and the therapists. DBT asks people to complete homework assignments, to role-play new ways of interacting with others, and to practice skills such as soothing yourself when upset. These skills are a crucial part of DBT and are taught in weekly lectures, reviewed in weekly homework groups, and referred to in nearly every group. The individual therapist helps the person to learn, apply, and master these skills.

Skills Training Modules

- Core Mindfulness – focusing skills
- Distress Tolerance – crisis survival skills
- Emotion Regulation – de-escalation skills
- Interpersonal Effectiveness – people skills

Core Mindfulness

Mindfulness allows me to be right here, right now, with no judgement – period. I can be present for those people in my life, under any and all circumstances, and be okay, no matter what. I would never, ever have believed that I could have that freedom and peace of mind in my life, but I do, today, and I am so grateful for it.

Mindfulness is not a matter of your mind controlling you, but you controlling your mind – not through explaining and solving but through experiencing and describing. Awareness plus acceptance of the current moment by simply focusing on one thing, without judgement, sounds so simple, and, trust me, with practice, it will become that for you. It is the ability to have full awareness of one's sensory and cognitive experience and to discern verbal descriptions of events, memories, and perceptions of events from each other.

Steps in Mindfulness

First, you will *observe*. Just notice what is taking place, and then *describe* and begin to put words to the experience. And, lastly, *participate* to become actively involved in the experience.

Using mindfulness, you will be able to calm yourself, better understand, and manage your emotions, re-centre, reflect, or train your brain to stay in the moment or be present.

Distress Tolerance

Dialectical behavior therapy emphasizes learning to bear pain skillfully, as it does with distress tolerance skills, which naturally develop from mindfulness skills. They have to do with the ability to accept, in a non-evaluative and non-judgmental fashion, both oneself and the current situation. Although the stance advocated here is a non-judgmental one, this does not mean that it is one of approval. Acceptance of reality is not approval of reality.

Distress tolerance behaviors are concerned with tolerating and surviving crises and with accepting life as it is in the moment. The four key components for distress tolerance are as follows:

1. Distracting
2. Self-soothing
3. Improving the moment
4. Focusing on pros and cons

One example of a distracting technique is ACCEPTS:

A is for activities and distracting oneself with healthy, enjoyable pursuits such as hobbies, exercise, and visiting with friends.

C is for contributing and doing things to help others, through volunteering or just a thoughtful gesture.

C is for comparing oneself to those less fortunate and finding reasons to be grateful.

E is for emotion; identifying the current, negative emotion and acting in an opposite manner, such as dancing or singing when one is feeling sad.

P is for pushing away by mentally leaving the current situation and focusing on something pleasant and unconnected to the present circumstances.

T is for thoughts and diverting one's attention from the negative feelings with unrelated and neural thoughts, such as counting items or doing a puzzle.

S is for sensations, and distracting oneself with physical sensations using multiple senses, like holding an ice cube, drinking a hot beverage, or enjoying a warm foot soak.

Emotional Regulation

People with BPD or who may be suicidal are typically emotionally intense and labile, frequently angry, intensely frustrated, depressed, and anxious. This suggests that people grappling with these concerns might benefit from help in learning to regulate their emotions. DBT skills for emotional regulation include:

- Learning to properly identify and label emotions
- Identifying obstacles to changing emotions
- Reducing vulnerability to an "emotional mind"
- Increasing positive emotional events
- Increasing mindfulness for current emotions

- Taking opposite action
- Applying distress tolerance techniques

Emotional regulation teaches how to manage difficult emotions and reduce suffering. One strategy for reducing emotional vulnerability is PLEASE MASTER:

PL represents taking care of your physical health and treating pain and/or illness.

E is for eating a balanced diet and avoiding excess sugar, fat, and caffeine.

A stands for avoiding alcohol and drugs, which only exacerbate emotional instability.

S represents getting regular and adequate sleep.

E is for getting regular exercise.

The MASTER part refers to daily activities that build confidence and competencies, with the goal of reducing emotional suffering while still feeling the emotions.

Interpersonal Effectiveness

Interpersonal effectiveness describes how we:

- Attend to relationships
- Balance priorities versus demands
- Balance the "wants" and "shoulds"
- Build a sense of mastery and self-respect

In order to increase your effectiveness in dealing with other people, you need to clarify what you want from the interaction and be as specific about that as you can by identifying what you need to do in order to get the results you want. One strategy for increasing interpersonal effectiveness is DEAR MAN:

Describe the current situation

Express your feelings and opinions

Assert yourself by asking for what you want, or by saying no

Reward the person – let them know what they will get out of it

Mindful of objectives without distraction (broken record technique, ignoring attacks)

Appear effective and competent (roleplay, use your acting skills)

Negotiate alternative solutions

Cognitive Behavioural Therapy (CBT)

CBT is based on the theory that much of how we feel is determined by what we think. Changing our cognition, our thoughts, and changing our behaviours are the two main components that make up CBT. Psychological problems are based, in part, on faulty or unhelpful ways of thinking and on learned patterns of unhelpful behavior. People suffering from psychological problems can learn better ways of coping with them, thereby relieving their symptoms and becoming more effective in their lives. CBT treatment usually involves efforts to change thinking patterns. These strategies might include learning to recognizing one's distortions in thinking that are creating problems, and then re-evaluating them while considering reality, gaining a better understanding of the behaviour and motivation of others, using problem-solving skills to cope with difficult situations, and learning to develop a greater sense of confidence in one's own abilities.

CBT treatment also usually involves efforts to change behavioral patterns. These strategies might include facing one's fears instead of avoiding them; using roleplaying to prepare for potentially problematic interactions with others and learning to calm one's mind and relax one's body, using mindfulness and grounding exercises. People with mental health issues often have inaccurate beliefs about themselves, their situations, and the world around them.

Common Cognitive Errors

Personalization

Personalization refers to relating negative events to oneself when there is no basis. An example of this is if someone doesn't respond to you, and you automatically assume that the person is upset with you when the truth is that the person's attention was distracted with another important situation that had nothing to do with you.

Dichotomous Thinking

Dichotomous thinking refers to all or nothing, black or white thinking and is usually detected when a person can generate only two choices in a situation. An example of this is if your boss doesn't schedule you to work your regular shift next week, and you automatically think that it is either because you are getting cut back in your hours or that you are in trouble for something when neither of these are correct, and you are not considering any other possible scenario to explain why you may have to switch shifts for the week.

Selective Abstraction

Selective abstraction refers to focusing only on certain aspects of a situation, usually the most negative. An example of this is when you are given feedback, both positive and negative, and you are only able to focus on the negative feedback and interpret it as a lack of support.

Magnification/Minimization

Magnification and minimization refer to distorting the importance of particular events. An example of this is doing well in college and wanting to go to medical school, but then receiving a D in a history class and becoming demoralized thinking that his lifelong dream to become a doctor is no longer possible.

Chapter 10

Step 7

Universal Power and Connection to Recovery Supports

"Faith is taking the first step when you don't see the whole staircase."

Martin Luther King Jr.

It's All in a Name – Or Is It?

There was a time in my life when it really did matter to me what "it" was called, and I certainly could not call *it* God. Nope, not happening. Because if, and that's a big *if*, there was a God, he wasn't a good one. If he was, he would not have let the terrible things that happened to me as a kid and a young adult happen – period.

Thankfully Marie, my Sponsor, assured me that I didn't have to have a God, or any other traditional anything in my life. I could choose whatever, or whoever, I wanted to have in my life as my own conception of a higher power, and that was a place I could agree to start from.

So how did I begin to allow spirituality to work in my life? Well, let me tell you. At first, it really was by "acting as if," because it certainly didn't feel natural or normal in any respect. And being honest, in the beginning it felt funny to communicate with my Creator in any way. When I started to pray, the only one I knew was the first prayer I learned when I was a little girl.

I worked weekly with Marie on my spirituality because like any muscle, without regular workouts it won't grow.

So, I practiced praying, I wrote letters to my Creator, and I talked to Creator anytime something was on my mind. It did get easier and more comfortable as time went on, but I didn't notice any big changes day-to-day, until I experienced a spiritual miracle.

I attended an AA campout for the first time in July 2009. I consciously prayed surrounded by a dozen other women in recovery around a campfire, at an impromptu gathering in the middle of the magnificent forest in a BC Provincial Park. I asked Creator to remove my addiction to alcohol. Thankfully and gratefully, I left there and returned home four days later feeling as though I had never been a drinker – my prayer had been answered. I could not understand the phenomenon, and it was not the last time I would experience this unbelievable event. More recently, I asked to have my addiction to nicotine taken from me, and it was. I have completely given up consuming all refined sugar, and it is as though I am not missing anything from my life – simply unexplainable. If it were not to have happened for me, I would have had difficulty believing in the stories myself – but I know my own truth. Like I've shared with you in this book, the three main requirements for success are being honest, openminded, and willing. Again, so much of what we learn, we are.

What is GOD or Goddess

A friend of mine in recovery introduced me to the concept of "**G**ood **O**rderly **D**irection (God)," a concept I love because it is a simple, but very effective way to manage and digest the concept of God at the beginning of one's spiritual journey. What I would like to do is start with an invitation for you to choose a concept of your liking. The main goal is to encourage you to build a connection with a power or purpose greater than yourself. It doesn't so much matter what you choose to connect to, what matters is your sense of connection to it. Feel free to choose Great Spirit, That Which Pulls Us Through, Jesus Christ (if you are a Christian), the compassionate Buddha, pure and undifferentiated Consciousness, or simply the Mystery.

Your recovery is a journey, and if you are able to allow some form of "Good Orderly Direction" as your roadmap, it will not only help keep you from getting lost, but it will help you resist taking uncharted detours or "shortcuts." You may find that you become less fearful and healthier than when you were viewing the world through the bars of an ego cage. Some people call it direction or long-term goals. Whatever it is for you, it helps you stay the course.

Write a New Ending That I Can Own

Once I had a chance to begin practicing the ability to catch my thoughts and then change them to become more positive ones, I eventually got to the ultimate place of peace – but that took some time and a few things happened along the way. As you may remember from earlier in my story, I shared with you how I had become lost when I was two and it was a pivotal, life changing moment for me in very destructive way. I have since been able to consciously rewrite that ending, and I can now go back in my mind's eye and reimagine that scene in a way that works for me to help heal that little girl who was so damaged by that event. This idea can also be the notion of reaching inward and comforting your inner child and embracing her. She may still be lost, hurt, damaged and alone, but now with your own love and comfort, you can go inside, embrace your small child, and lead her back to the safety of your arms. Your heart will rewrite a different ending for her too – one that will make her happy, safe, loved, and secure.

What is Buddhism

About 2500 years ago, a prince named Siddhartha Gautama began to question his sheltered, luxurious life in a palace. He left the palace and saw four sights: a sick man, an old man, a dead man, and a monk. These sights are said to have shown him that even a prince cannot escape illness, suffering, and death. The sight of the monk lead Siddhartha to leave his life as a prince and become a wandering holy man, seeking the answers to questions like "Why must people suffer?" and "What is the cause of suffering?"

Siddhartha spent many years doing religious practices such as praying, meditating, and fasting until he finally understood the basic truths of life. This realization occurred after sitting under a Poplar-fig tree in Bodh Gaya, India, for many days in deep meditation. He gained enlightenment, or nirvana, and was given the title of Buddha, which means Enlightened One.

Buddha discovered the Three Universal Truths and Four Noble Truths, which he then taught to people for the next forty-five years. His Three Universal Truths were:

1. Everything in life is impermanent and always changing.

2. Because nothing is permanent, a life based on possessing things or persons doesn't make you happy.
3. There is no eternal, unchanging soul, and "self" is just a collection of changing characteristics or attributes.

His Four Noble Truths were:

1. Human life has a lot of suffering.
2. The cause of suffering is greed.
3. There is an end to suffering.
4. The way to end suffering is to follow the Middle Path.

Buddha then taught people not to worship him as a god. He said they should take responsibility for their own lives and actions. He taught that the Middle Way was the way to nirvana. The Middle Way meant not leading a life of luxury and indulgence but also not one of too much fasting and hardship. There are eight guides for following the Middle path.

The Eightfold Path

1. Right understanding and viewpoint (based on the Four Noble Truths)
2. Right values and attitude (compassion rather than selfishness)
3. Right speech (don't tell lies, avoid harsh, abusive speech, and avoid gossip)
4. Right action (help others, live honestly, don't harm living things, and take care of the environment)
5. Right work (do something useful and avoid jobs which harm others)

6. Right effort (encourage good, helpful thoughts, and discourage unwholesome destructive thoughts)
7. Right mindfulness (be aware of what you feel, think, and do)
8. Right meditation (keep a calm mind and practice meditation which leads to nirvana)

What Is Meditation?

Meditation is an essential practice to most Buddhists. Buddhists look within themselves for the truth and understanding of Buddha's teachings. They seek enlightenment, or nirvana, in this way. Nirvana is freedom from needless suffering and being fully alive and present in one's life. It is not a state that can really be described in words – it goes beyond words.

Meditation means focusing the mind to achieve an inner stillness that leads to a state of enlightenment. Meditation takes many forms:

- It can be sitting quietly beside a beautiful arrangement of rocks, contemplating beauty.
- It can be practicing a martial art such as karate or aikido, since they require mental and physical control and strong concentration.
- It can mean focusing on a riddle such as "What is the sound of one hand clapping?"
- It can be contemplating a haiku or short poem that captures a moment in time.
- It can be in a meditation room of a monastery.
- It can involve chanting.

- It can involve the use of a mandala to focus your attention on the invisible point at the center of interlocking triangles.
- It can involve quietly noticing one's breath as it goes in and out.
- It can happen anywhere at any time.

The Five Precepts

Even though each form of Buddhism took on its own identity, all Buddhists follow a set of guidelines for daily life called the Five Precepts. These are:

1. Do not harm or kill living things
2. Do not take things unless they are freely given
3. Lead a decent life
4. Do not speak unkindly or tell lies
5. Do not abuse drugs or drink alcohol

Prayers and Poems

To help you in finding your spirituality, looking inward, and meditating, I've compiled a list of prayers and poems that have been helpful in my healing journey. Feel free to use these on your healing journey, as well.

Indigenous People's Cherokee Indian Healing Prayer

Great Mystery, teach me how
to trust my heart, my mind,

My intuition, my inner knowing,
the senses of my body,

The blessings of my spirit.

Teach me to trust these things
so that I may enter my

Sacred Space and love beyond my fear,
and thus walk in

Balance with passing of each glorious sun.

The Knots Prayer

Dear God
Please untie the knots that are in my mind,
my heart and my life.
Remove the have nots, the can nots and
the do nots
that I have in my mind.
Erase the will nots, may nots,
might nots that may find a home in my heart.
Release me from the could nots, would nots and
should nots that obstruct my life.
And most of all,
Dear God,
I ask that you remove from my mind, my heart
and my life all of the 'am nots'
that I have allowed to hold me back, especially
the thought
that I am not good enough.
Amen

Prayer for Health

*O' Sacred Heart of God, I come to ask
for the gift of restored health,*

*That I may serve you more faithfully and love you
more sincerely than in the past.*

*I want to be well and strong if it is your will
and rebound to your glory.*

*If in your divine wisdom I am to be restored
to health and strength of mind, body, and spirit,*

*I will strive to show my gratitude by a constant
and faithful service rendered to you.*

The Prayer That Started It All for Me

*Now I lay me down to sleep, I pray the lord my soul to
keep. If I should die before I wake, I pray the lord my
soul to take...thank you God, for my life, my breath
and my sobriety, thank you for the good, the bad and
the indifferent, thank for everything that happened
today. Thank you for gifting me my loves, Brianna
and my fur baby Moo, who never leave my side and
show me every day what unconditional love and
acceptance is. Thank you for allowing me to be
present for my mom and dad, so I can be there for
them as best I can.*

This Is Your Awakening by S. Carroll

The Awakening

There comes a time in your life when you finally get it... When in the midst of all your fears and insanity you stop dead in your tracks and somewhere the voice inside your head cries out "ENOUGH! Enough fighting and crying or struggling to hold on." And, like a child quieting down after a blind tantrum, your sobs begin to subside, you shudder once or twice, you blink back your tears, and through a mantle of wet lashes you begin to look at the world from a new perspective.

...This is your awakening.

Recovery Support and Tools

In addition to the prayers and poems that have helped me in my recovery, AA has been instrumental in providing me spiritual mottos that have helped me succeed in healing. I've shared some of the mottos below.

First Things First

We are often the type of people who lack order in our lives, so here is an orderly method of doing things which I have found greatly helpful. When we are confused, let us say "First Things First" and put the most important matters in first place, and in second, third, and so on. This tool helps us to think logically.

Live and Let Live

If we follow our principles, we have to respect other people's opinions, allowing the person to live his/her own life without your judgement. When we feel resentment creeping in, let us say to ourselves "Live and Let Live." It may save us an embarrassing situation.

Easy Does It

This tool can be used many times a day if you are prone to panic. Oldtimers have said there were many times in the early days of alcoholics anonymous when this motto saved them from taking a drink. Some members have used this during a relapse from panic. If you say "Easy Does It" it gives you time to think. Sometimes this is all you need to avoid a mistake.

Keep an Open Mind

To balance our thinking, your mind must be open to new ideas. If you are on the defensive and feel the need to protect yourself, your mind is shut. Today we strive to understand people rather than demanding that they understand us. There is a saying in AA which is that our minds should not be so open that an idea would coast right through. Another AA quip tells us "take the cotton out of your ears and put it in your mouth".

Prayer Changes Things

When things are going well, for many of us, we forget prayer. Once again, you have to be reminded that prayer has changed your life. It has been said that prayer moves mountains

– didn't it move a mountain for you? This reminds me of another motto, "Lest we forget."

Know Thyself

Who am I? What am I? Where am I going? Why? These are questions we have thought about for years – now through our program, we are learning the truth about ourselves. There is another quotation, "To Thine Own Self Be True." You can do great things if you understand "me," know me, and be true to me. The most important person in your life – me – is the only person you can change. Let it begin with me.

The Importance of Human Connection

What do you do from day to day to care for yourself? What about your social connections?

According the Canadian Mental Health Association, loneliness is on the rise, and a lack of human connection can be more harmful to your health than obesity, smoking, and high blood pressure.

In today's age, we live busy lives, trying to strike a balance between work, school, hobbies, self-care, and more. Often, our social connections fall by the wayside. But connecting with others is more important than you might think. Social connection can lower anxiety and depression, help regulate emotions, lead to higher self-esteem and empathy, and improve your immune system. By neglecting your need to connect, you put your health at risk.

The reality is that we're living in a time of true disconnection. While technology seems to connect us more than ever, the screens around us disconnect us from nature, from ourselves, and from others. Wi-Fi alone isn't enough to fulfill your social needs – you need face-to-face interaction to thrive. Technology should be enhancing our connection to others, not replacing it.

Our inherent need for human connection doesn't mean that every introvert must become a social butterfly. Having human connection can look different for each person. And if you're not sure where to start in finding meaningful connection, that's okay. Here are some ideas to help you out:

- Join a new club, or try out a group activity
- Reach out to an old friend you've lost touch with
- Volunteer for a cause you care about
- Eat lunch in a communal space
- Introduce yourself to your neighbors
- Ask someone for help when you need it
- Do a random act of kindness

If you're feeling lonely, know you're not the only one. And that you don't have to live in isolation. We live in a world with over seven billion people, and we all need connection.

Unconditional Love of and Connection to a Pet

I really can't overemphasize the importance and value of having a pet of any sort, whether it walks, has four or two feet, fins or feathers, scales or spines, swims or slithers, or has a shell. This is especially the case for those of us with a huge fear of abandonment or issues with identity, self-esteem, validation, connection, and a desire to feel loved. A pet can be an instant prescription for 24/7 love that will do your heart and soul good all day long, every day of the week.

I am blessed to have a dog by the name of Moo – he is a cross between a Shih-Tzu and a Japanese Chin. He is eleven years old now, and I don't know what I would do every day without Moo's unconditional love, acceptance, and companionship. He is an ongoing source of entertainment and always gives me a reason to smile and laugh from my belly. I couldn't imagine how I would have survived the long, lonely days and nights without him, and thank goodness I do not have to. Here's to my much-loved gift from God above for always showing me unconditional love and keeping me in the here and now.

Connections – Healthy Belonging

There is also importance in building healthy romantic connections. However, when building these relations there are important guidelines one should follow. The characteristics of healthy belonging for the individual include:

- Experiencing both oneness with and separateness from a partner
- Being able to bring out the best qualities in a partner
- Accepting endings and enjoying solitude
- Experiencing openness to change and exploration
- Experiencing true intimacy and welcome closeness
- Feeling the freedom to honestly for what is wanted
- Experience receiving and giving in the same way
- Not attempting to control or change the other person
- Encouraging self-sufficiency of partners

- Accepting limitations of self and partners
- Accepting commitment and not seeking uncondi-
tional love
- Expressing feelings spontaneously and affirming
equality of self and your partner
- Have a high self-esteem and welcome vulnerability

Chapter 11

Step 8

Depend on Yourself

> "Daring to set boundaries is about having the courage to love ourselves, even when we risk disappointing others."
>
> Brene Brown

Learning How to Say "Enough Is Enough"

I was taught an invaluable life lesson, although at the time I was unaware that schooling was underway – the best kind of learning indeed.

I had just embarked on my first weekend AA campout, a couple hour's drive from home, and was ready to finally surrender to sobriety after months of failed attempts and slips. I was prepared to do whatever I had to in order to stay sober. I was also about to realize, at thirty-eight years of age, how "loose" my boundaries were. They were virtually non-existent at that time. I truly had no idea that up until that point, I let people walk all over me. While this expression is not usually used in a literal sense, in the story I am about to share, I mean that I literally let someone walk all over me without so much as a word.

There I was, in the middle of a beautiful provincial park campground on Vancouver Island, in a mountainous, coastal region of British Columbia, Canada. A place of breathtaking scenery, with pristine forests, rivers, and lakes. I had settled in at my campsite, and feeling a little restless, decided to go for a walk until I found my intended destination – my Sponsor Marie's RV and campsite. Standing under the RV canopy, in the process of rolling it out, was her hubby, John. I offered to help him, but as usual, he had it all in hand, so I stood and watched as the rest of their outdoor area sprang to life with beautiful cushions, lively mats, and twinkle lights to offset the darkness moving in.

Later, I was discussing with John, an addictions counselor and in recovery himself, the difficulties I was having with my marriage, staying sober, and establishing limits. It all seemed too much, and I didn't know where to start. John approached me and asked me if I wanted his help with it, to which I replied, "Yes, please!" At that, John continued forward and stepped on my toes on my right foot. He just stood there looking at me straight in the eyes for about thirty to forty-five seconds, and then he stepped away. I thought it was a bit strange, and stranger yet a minute later, when he did it *again*. Then he asked me if I liked him stepping on my toes. I said, "No, I do not." He stepped off, and I could not believe it when for the third time, he actually stepped on my toes again, and this time, he leaned his face into mine, his nose almost touching mine, and had the nerve to say to me, "Do you want to me to be stepping on your toes now?" I said, "No, John, I don't want you to be stepping on my toes right now."

With that, John gave me the biggest smile I had ever seen on his face, and he stepped off my toes. At this point, I'm still unaware of the lesson he was teaching me – it was literally right in my face, but until he said to me, "Julie, how come you can't ask me to get off your toes? Why do you think that you aren't comfortable saying that to me, knowing that I shouldn't be standing on your toes?"

I had no response. I actually believed it was okay for someone to do something that caused me discomfort, and that I should remain silent and uncomfortable rather than stand up for myself and say "*hey*, you are violating my space, you are hurting my toes, and I want to you stop what you are doing to me now." In other words, I had to establish clear, healthy, and necessary boundaries for myself, which I had none of at that point. What an incredible and valuable lesson to have been taught so effectively and lovingly that I, at the age of thirty-eight, didn't have boundaries. Later in this chapter, I will discuss the types of boundaries, as well as how to begin building the foundation to establish crucial limits in relationships, as the construction of boundaries will be a lifelong task.

Oxygen Mask

How many of you have ever flown on a commercial airliner? You'll recall that after the cabin doors are locked and the plane is moving towards the runway, the flight attendants will proceed to line the aisle checking the overhead bins and that your luggage is properly stowed away under the seat in front of you. Once they've done that, the safety announcement and instructions commence, and then an oxygen mask is demonstrated. The very next thing that is said is *really* important: in the event of an emergency, if you are travelling with a child, an elderly person, or another vulnerable person, it is of great importance that you ensure that you put your oxygen mask on first. If something should happen, and you don't have your mask on, there is a possibility that you will not be able to assist anyone else. The lesson here is to make sure that you take care of your needs first so that you can assist others, especially your loved ones, when they need you. If you aren't looking after yourself, you won't have anything for them when they truly require your assistance.

Self-Care Is How You Reclaim Your Power

Simply stated, it is in the act of taking care of yourself that you will begin the process of reclaiming your power. Once you have established a routine of taking care of your essential self-care needs, it is through this process that a miraculous thing happens. Over time, the connection will grow to re-establish the relationship between your mind, body, and spirit. As this process is underway, you will begin to feel a shift within yourself, and you will begin reclaiming your power, and, ultimately, your ability to like and eventually love yourself. For some of you, myself included, it will be a brand-new feeling that you may never have imagined was possible, and certainly may never have felt before. It is through the small acts of kindness towards yourself that you end up receiving such huge rewards that can shift and propel you into new dimensions of thoughts and feelings you never dreamt possible.

You Don't Know What You Don't Know
Gluten Intolerance

What you eat everyday can very negatively impact how your system functions. Each person's system has varying intolerances and tendencies. From the food sensitivity test-ing I had done, I learned that, among other things, I was gluten intolerant. That meant that everything I ate which contained gluten, essentially everything containing flour, had an enzyme in it that my body could not digest, and, as a result, my body's natural defense mechanism was causing inflammation. For instance, every piece of toast that I put jam on, would cause massive swelling in both my stom-ach, brain, and other tissues in my body, which could, and likely was, causing pain and discomfort for me. All because I introduced both gluten and sugar into my fragile eco system that was never designed to process gluten or refined sugar, and as a result, my body's natural response was to become inflamed. I was being greatly impacted and affected.

You may have noticed that a lot of diseases end in "itis", which simply means inflammation or inflamed. For example, sinusitis is chronic inflammation of the sinus cavity, and tendonitis is the inflammation of the tendons. Having said that, what happens to those of us with gluten intolerance is that initially, the inflammation is limited mainly to the gastro-systems. However, over time, the body's tolerance lessens, and the effects can become more severe, resulting in widespread symptomatic issues such as brain fog, chronic fatigue, extreme sensitivities, difficulty concentrating, and increased emotionality. A large portion of the population is not aware that this is taking place in their bodies, or that inflammation caused by gluten could be affecting them at all. It was only after I eliminated it from my diet completely that I was able to understand and feel the difference it made in my body. It changed, not only, how I felt about the food

I was eating, but also my understanding of how the food I was eating was affecting me.

The best suggestion I can give you is if you are curious, what have you got to lose? Inflammation and pain? Eliminate gluten from your diet for a week. I'm willing to bet that you'll notice a difference after a few days, and the proof will be in how good you feel without it in your system.

A quote on the effects of gluten from Food Renegade: "undigested gluten proteins hang out in your intestines and are treated by our bodies like foreign invaders, causing irritation in the gut and flattening the microvilli along the small intestinal wall lessening its ability to absorb the nutrients from the food we eat. In addition, it causes horrible pain, vomiting, and diarrhea after gluten is consumed. If the symptoms are so intense, it may go undetected and can lead to further issues such as autoimmune diseases, which can be exhausting, frustrating, and overall very uncomfortable to say the least."

The most common symptoms are as follows:

- Stomach pain – you know what they say, listen to your gut
- Dizziness – brain fog, disorientation, and feeling off balance
- Mood swings – unexplainably irritable, anxious, or upset
- Chronic migraine – typically occurring thirty to sixty minutes after eating and can lead to blurry vision
- Itchy skin – inward inflammation reveals itself outwardly through skin conditions like eczema and psoriasis

- Fibromyalgia – avoiding gluten can alleviate fibromy-algia according to many health professionals such as Medicine Net rheumatology expert Dr. Alex Shikhman
- Chronic Fatigue – since your mind is up and down, you'll feel tired and exhausted and wake up after a full night sleep still feeling drained, as your body is always inflamed
- Lactose intolerance – gluten and dairy intolerance go hand in hand, and it can be surprising; this is based on a type of sugar found in dairy products that triggers gluten intolerance and adds to the symptoms

For more information on gluten intolerance visit www.littlethings.com/signs-of-gluten-intolerance.

White Sugar

In my opinion, and backed by many health professionals, sugar is a food item to be avoided when someone has issues with inflammation, such as arthritis or chronic pain, not to mention mental health issues. When I was able to finally say goodbye to sugar, which was not a happy farewell but a very sad parting of company, my pain level dropped so significantly that I was astonished. My doctor had told me that I could expect it would be reduced by as much as 50 percent, but I would say that it was even greater than that most days. However, I do notice that on days when my stress levels are high, my pain levels are higher also.

When looking at the impact of sugar on mental health, it is believed and understood that sugar can cause obe-sity and contributes to widespread inflammation. It can also contribute to poor dental health and lead to diabetes. Many people don't stop and think that it can also have a very detrimental impact on mental health, but now conclusive research shows that it does have a negative impact on mood, learning, and the quality of life you live. As importantly, the research shows that sugar, honey, maple syrup, corn syrup, and molasses can have a detrimental impact on mental well-being due to the rapid fluctuation of blood sugar, which can worsen mood disorders and can lead to an increased risk of depression.

Although sugar does not increase your risk of anxiety, it can worsen the symptoms and weaken the body's response to stress. By minimizing the amount of sugar, you can lessen the severity of anxiety symptoms improve your mood and the body's ability to cope with stress. There's also a growing amount of evidence of the addictive potential of sugar, not unlike drugs, as both flood the brain with "feel good" chemical dopamine. So, it would stand to reason that sugar can affect how much we learn and remember. In studies and tests, it is shown that rats forgot how to find their way out of a maze after six weeks of drinking a fructose solution, and insulin resistance from a higher sugar diet can damage communications between brain cells involved in learning and memory formation. What has become the norm in North American society regarding the consumption of sugar is much greater than what our minds and bodies were designed to process. And now that we are aware that it plays a significant role in both physical and mental health, grappling with mental illness is difficult enough without adding more obstacles into the mix, my suggestion is to make the situation easier by eliminating sugar. Don't fret because there are lots of great things you can replace it with and lots of people once over the hump, don't miss it at all.

Replace any foods with added sugar in your diet and read your labels carefully. Many foods you wouldn't suspect have added sugars are sweetened with them such as pasta sauces, salad dressings, and condiments sauces like ketchups and relishes etc. If you're craving a sweet snack, eat fruit. Cut down or, better yet, cut out all sodas or fruit juices all together and replace them with water or herbal teas. Any diet sodas and artificial sweeteners are not a good option as they have other health concerns in the artificial composition which make them up. Flavoured yogurts are very high in sugar, so instead buy plain yogurt and add a dash of vanilla and fresh fruit to have a bowl of delicious, refreshing, enjoyment.

I was truly amazed when I gave up sugar as I watched thirty pounds melt off my frame in the next three months without any other effort made on my part to try and lose weight whatsoever! My pain levels were reduced significantly from the arthritis and fibromyalgia, as well, which was my main motivation for cutting out the sugar in the first place. Now that's what I call a win-win-win!

Understanding What Co-dependency Is and How It Affects Your Relationships and Behaviours

Co-dependence is a condition that stifles your true self, your child within. It results from and contributes to all parental conditions in a dysfunctional or alcoholic family.

It can be defined as any suffering and/or dysfunction that is associated with or results from focusing on the needs and behaviour of others, to the exclusion of your own needs. Anne Wilson Sheaffer says in her book *Co-dependence: Misunderstood – Mistreated* that codependents can be so focused upon or preoccupied with important people and others' lives that they neglect their true self. This can lead to a process of nonliving, which is progressive.

Endemic in ordinary humankind, co-dependence can mimic, be associated with, and aggravate many conditions. It develops from turning your responsibility for your life and happiness over to your ego and to other people.

Development of Co-dependence

The genesis of co-dependence begins by the repression of your observations, feelings, and reactions. Many often-become parents and eventually begin to invalidate these often-crucial internal cues.

As a result of the denial and the secrets they keep, with the focus being on others, they deny and stifle their child within. That is because they still often have feelings of hurt and will start feeling and become increasingly numb and tolerant of emotional pain. They are unable to grieve their everyday losses to completion. All of this blocks their growth and development in the mental, emotional, and spiritual aspects of their being. But they have a desire to contact and know their true selves. They learned that quick fixes such as compulsive behaviors will allow them to catch glimpses of their true selves and will let off some of the tension. However, if the compulsive behaviour is distractive to them and others, they will feel shame that will result in a lower self-esteem. At this point they may begin to feel more and more out of control and try to compensate with the need to control even more. They may end up diluted and hurt and often project their pain onto others.

Their attention has now built to such an extent that they may develop stress related illness manifested as aches and pains and often dysfunction of one or more body organs. They are now in an advance state of co-dependence and may progressively deteriorate so that they may experience one or more of extreme mood swings and difficulty with intimate relationships. For those of us who are attempting to recover from alcoholism or another chemical dependency or another chronic condition or illness dependency may seriously interfere.

In my case, as I began to deal with my alcoholism, my need to control got worse to the point that it became unmanageable. I was controlling everything and everybody in my life down to the smallest detail and degree to try and have some manageability in my life and was failing at all of it. In fact, it was only making things worse, but I didn't realize it at the time. It's only been in recent years that my daughter and I have been able to talk about it, and she's been comfortable sharing her experiences with me that has allowed me to realize the degree and depth of my controlling nature during that period. I realize the co-dependency I felt in my relationships were at the root of the crazy making and the controlling behaviour I was exhibiting before I began making progress in my recovery from co-dependency and BPD.

Co-dependency is typically discussed in the context of substance use, where one person is abusing the substance, and he or she depends on the other person to supply money, food, or shelter. But, according to Jonathan Becker, DO, assistant professor of clinical psychiatry at Vanderbilt University in Nashville, Tennessee, dependency is much broader than that.

"Co-dependency can be defined as any relationship in which two people become so invested in each other that they can't function independently anymore," Dr. Becker says. "Your mood, happiness, and identity are defined by the other person. In a codependent relationship, there is usually one person who is more passive and can't make decisions for themselves, and a more dominant personality who gets some reward and satisfaction from controlling the other person and making decisions about how they will live." Signs of co-dependency include:

- Having difficulty making decisions in a relationship
- Having difficulty identifying your feelings
- Having difficulty communicating in a relationship
- Valuing the approval of others more than you value yourself
- Lacking trust in yourself and having poor self-esteem
- Having fears of abandonment or an obsessive need for approval
- Having an unhealthy dependence on relationships, even at your own cost
- Having an exaggerated sense of responsibility for the actions of others

Boundaries

Huge growth started happening for me when I started checking and correcting myself instead of blaming other people, especially my family, for being stuck. I really started paying attention to the right people and things and taking care of myself, and I began getting my power back by being fully responsible for myself and for my life, with no more excuses and no more wasted time living in the past.

When I say yes to you, I am saying no to me. Many of us can't say no and don't realize that it is not only okay to say no, but it is necessary for our own best interests to do so. In fact, "no" is a complete sentence. Saying no will allow you to be more fully present for others when you are first taking care of your needs. You can only give to others when you have something to give. We are so busy being busy and overscheduling our lives, these days, that we are missing the mark, falling behind, and end up feeling like we are failing at everything. Instead, take things in manageable "bite-size" pieces and this will allow you to make time for what's top priority for you, and then you can determine what time you have left to assist others. We don't have to disappoint others, when we do our planning first.

Below is a list of guidelines to help you in setting your own boundaries:

- It's not my job to fix others
- It's okay to say no
- It's not my job to take responsibility for others
- I don't have to anticipate the needs for others
- Nobody has to agree with me

- I am responsible for my own happiness
- I have a right to my own feelings
- I have a right to express my needs honestly
- I am enough

Boundary Statements

- Boundaries are dividers between you and others.
- If someone is mad at you, you don't have to feel guilty.
- If someone doesn't like you, it doesn't mean you are unlikeable.
- If someone asks you to do something, you don't have to say yes.
- If someone thinks you should do something, it doesn't mean it is the right choice for you.
- If someone is unhappy, it doesn't mean you have to be too.
- If someone has a different opinion, it doesn't mean yours is wrong.

Name Your Limits

According to psychologist Dana Gionta, PhD, it's important to identify your physical, emotional, mental, and spiritual limits. Consider what you can tolerate and accept and what makes you feel uncomfortable or stressed. "Those feelings help us identify what our limits are."

Tune into Your Feelings

Gionta has observed two key feelings that are red flags or cues that you're letting go of your boundaries: discomfort and resentment. She suggested thinking of these feelings on a continuum from one to ten with six to ten being the higher zone. If you're at the higher end of this continuum, during an interaction or in a situation, Gionta suggests asking yourself what is causing that. What is it about this interaction, or the person's expectation that is bothering you?

Resentment usually "comes from being taken advantage of or not appreciated." It's often a sign that you're pushing yourself either beyond your own limits because you feel guilty (and want to be a good daughter or wife, for instance), or someone else is imposing their expectations, views or values on you.

Gionta says, "When someone acts in a way that makes you feel uncomfortable, that's a cue to us they may be violating or crossing a boundary."

Be Direct

With some people, maintaining healthy boundaries doesn't require a direct and clear-cut dialogue. Usually, this is the case if people are similar in their communication styles, views, personalities, and general approach to life. They'll "approach each other similarly."

With others, such as those who have a different personality or cultural background, you'll need to be more direct about your boundaries. Consider the following example: "one person feels [that] challenging someone's opinions is a healthy way of communicating," but to another person this feels disrespectful and tense.

However, Gionta believes there are other times you might need to be direct. For instance, in a romantic relationship, time can become a boundary issue. Partners might need to talk about how much time they need to maintain their sense of self and how much time to spend together.

Give Yourself Permission

Gionta identifies fear, guilt, and self-doubt as big potential pitfalls. You might fear the other person's response if you set and enforce your boundaries. You might feel guilty by speaking up or saying no to a family member. Many believe that they should be able to cope with a situation or say yes because they're a good daughter or son, even though they "feel drained or taken advantage of." You might wonder if you even deserve to have boundaries in the first place.

Boundaries aren't just a sign of a healthy relationship; they're a sign of self-respect. So, give yourself the permission to set boundaries and work to preserve them.

Practice Self-Awareness

Again, boundaries are all about homing in on your feelings and honoring them. If you notice yourself slipping and not sustaining your boundaries, Gionta suggests asking yourself what has changed? Consider, "What I am doing or [what is] the other person doing?" or "What is the situation eliciting that's making me resentful or stressed?" Then, mull over your options and ask yourself, "What am I going to do about the situation? What do I have control over?"

Consider Your Past and Present

According to Gionta, how you were raised along with your role in your family can become additional obstacles in setting and preserving boundaries. If you held the role of caretaker, you learned to focus on others, letting yourself be drained emotionally or physically. Ignoring your own needs might have become the norm for you. Think about the people you surround yourself with. "Are the relationships reciprocal?" Is there a healthy give and take?

Beyond relationships, your environment might be unhealthy, too. For instance, if your workday is eight hours a day, but your co-workers stay for at least ten to eleven hours, "there's an implicit expectation to go above and beyond" at work. It can be challenging being the only one or one of a few trying to maintain healthy boundaries. Again, this is where tuning into your feelings and needs and honoring them becomes critical.

Make Self-Care a Priority
Gionta helps her clients make self-care a priority, which involves giving themselves permission to put themselves first. When we do this, "our need and motivation to set boundaries becomes stronger". Self-care also means recognizing the importance of your feelings and honoring them. These feelings serve as "important cues about our wellbeing and about what makes us happy and unhappy."

Putting yourself first also gives you the "energy, peace of mind and positive outlook to be more present with others and be there for them." When you're in a better place, you can be a better wife, mother, husband, co-worker, or friend.

Seek Support
If you're having a hard time with boundaries, "seek some support, whether [that's a] support group, church, counseling, coaching or good friends". With friends or family, you

can even make "it a priority with each other to practice setting boundaries together [and] hold each other accountable."

Gionta recommends considering seeking support through resources, too. She likes the following books: *The Art of Extreme Self-Care: Transform Your Life One Month at a Time* and *Boundaries in Marriage* (along with several books on boundaries by the same authors).

Be Assertive

Of course, you know that it's not enough to create boundaries; you actually have to follow through. Gionta surmises that even though you know, intellectually, that people aren't mind readers, you still expect others to know what hurts you. Since they don't, it's important to assertively communicate with the other person when that person crosses a boundary. Gionta recommends, in a respectful way, letting the other person know what is bothersome to you so you can work together to address it.

Start Small

Like any new skill, assertively communicating your boundaries takes practice. Gionta suggests starting with a small boundary that isn't threatening to you, and then incrementally increasing it to more challenging boundaries. "Build upon your success, and [at first] try not to take on something that feels overwhelming." As Gionta says, "Setting boundaries takes courage, practice, and support." And remember that it's a skill you can master.

Anger

Anger is your body's response to a perceived provocation, so what do you do about it? First of all, start by thanking it. Yes, that's right, thank it. Anger is your body's way of saying that there *may* be a threat of some sort, and your body allows you to make a choice about the best way to use your energy to determine how to respond to the threat. It is giving you the opportunity to act.

When you're angry, and in all situations, I would encourage you to consider the other person's point of view to see if you can understand why that person did or said what was done or said. I like to operate with the assumption of best intentions always, and then I don't find myself questioning anyone's motives. If, on the other hand, their motives become apparent during the conversation – the facts will always prevail. Two seemingly opposing viewpoints can both be right rather than someone having to be wrong. Make lemonade. Try to find the good that came out of it. How did you emerge stronger? How could it have been worse? What do you have to be grateful for? Lessons can always be learned. Take a walk. Anger kicks up your fight or flight hormones. Use up some of that energy to get grounded.

HALT Method

When you get angry, stop and use HALT: ask yourself if you are **H**ungry, **A**ngry, **L**onely, or **T**ired. If you are any of these things, address them right away, and you will be less likely to find yourself in challenging situations. Common sense goes a long way here, so if you are hungry, take the time to eat something as nutritious as possible. Recognize that a chocolate bar, for instance, will give you immediate gratification, but will likely lead you to a sugar crash. On the other hand, a handful of fresh veggies and hummus will be both satisfying and better for your system overall.

Healthy anger has value so long as it is properly vented, but repression of anger can cause more damage when not released and dealt with properly. I encourage you to take a moment first, and look at what needs to be done before you react and determine: a) does the situation need to be changed, b) can you do something about it, or c) can you change your response to the situation (i.e. let it go, accept it, etc.)? Only then are you ready to make an informed decision about how best to proceed. If you are feeling lonely, reach out and call a friend, and if the first one you phone isn't available for a chat or a visit, keep dialing until someone is. It is important to stay connected, especially when things aren't going so well. And last, but certainly not least, are you tired? You may not realize how much more vulnerable and fragile you feel, I know I certainly do, when you are without proper sleep. I lose the ability to manage key elements of my life as easily as I can when I am rested. I have experienced this enough firsthand to know how crucial it is that I maintain a consistent sleep schedule and hygiene.

Write it Down and Talk Again Later

If you are angry with someone, it may be best to write out your thoughts and get together later to discuss the situation when both of you are calm. When you are angry, the adrenaline can keep you from seeing the big picture. Additionally, when you walk away, you can avoid being impulsive. When you write things down, you can get everything out and then the hurtful, aggressive remarks will be less likely to be part of the exchange. This will also reduce the likelihood of severing relationships, as it gives you a chance to cool off and rethink before you say something in the heat of the moment that you are not able to take back once it has been said.

Work on Your Self-Esteem

Many anger triggers have to do with fearing rejection, being judged, failing in some way, or not being able to change someone else's opinion of you, whether it is real or imagined. A positive self-esteem allows you to be okay with the fact that nobody will like you all the time, and that is okay! Remember to focus on your square foot of space only – you can not change anyone else, or even just their opinion for that matter!

Tale of Two Wolves

Years and years ago, my dad shared with me a story that a Shaman he had met at a sweat lodge told him. He told him that inside each of us, there are two wolves. One is a black wolf who is filled with hurt, anger, jealousy, greed, resentment, and inferiority. The other is a white wolf who is helpful, filled with joy, peace, love, acceptance, kindness, and truth. The wolf that will flourish and survive is the one that you give your attention to – the one that you feed. Choose wisely which one you will be feeding and giving your attention to.

Chapter 12

Step 9

Elevate Yourself

"Before everything else, getting ready is the secret of success."

Henry Ford

Golden Rules to Survive and Thrive with BPD

I am blessed to have such a strong and decent moral compass from which I derived these golden rules. I live my life by them and in most cases, they eliminate the need for guess work, for which I am very thankful and grateful. I use the following list to help me navigate day-to-day when I have even the slightest conflict about how to conduct myself and make decisions. I invite you to use any or all of these as well, and you may find, as I do, that it makes it so much simpler to understand what the right path is when emotions and feelings come charging in, complicating things. It also takes the personalness out of it, so that I don't feel bad about my decisions afterward because I know with certainty the "why" behind my decision; therefore, I am much less prone to second guessing or overthinking. For this overthinker, this is a great tool to utilize. No need to analyze, just see below.

Do the Next Right Thing, and the Next Right Thing Happens

This one is self-explanatory and works no matter what the circumstances are – the more complicated they are, the more helpful it is. It takes the guess work out, along with the emotions, mixed feelings, and the personal side of things. Something that has tripped me up is when I don't know what my role is, especially in a codependent relationship dynamic. The expression states clearly that if I do the next right thing, the next right thing will happen, but it doesn't say when or how. What's required is patience combined with a belief that it will happen, and you can guarantee your future success. Trust in that – I do. And I have experienced, time and time again, it works! My personal version of the Law of Attraction.

Life Doesn't Get Better by Chance, It Gets Better by Change

Over the last ten years that I have been on Facebook, I have only posted one quote to describe myself and it is the one above. Why did I choose this one quote? Because of how often I hear people saying that they are unhappy with their current state of affairs, and yet, they don't seem to see that the only way things will get any better is if they are willing to do something to change their situation. Things won't improve just by thinking about how unhappy you are – that is guaranteed to make them worse. The situation will only change when you, yourself, begin to affect changes in your way of thinking. Then, from your thinking to your actions to make the necessary change will bring forth the desired end result, which is a change in circumstances to improve the overall quality of life that you have been desiring. Makes sense, right?

Is Any Good Going to Come from This?

Again, such a huge one when it comes to deciding whether to engage in a situation or not, and it allows me to avoid the "yeah, but" syndrome that used to plague me. When something crosses my path today, I always do the litmus test by asking "is any good going to come from me saying this, doing this, writing this, sharing this, repeating this, etc." – you get my drift. If the answer is not a clear *yes*, then my answer is a clear *no*! It takes a lot of the guess work out of tricky situations, especially when there are different dynamics at play, or when people try to influence your decision, possibly confusing your moral compass. By asking myself this question, no matter what another person's question or opinion may be, it always helps me to become really clear with my decision and subsequent confident answer.

Would You Rather Be Right, or Be Happy?

This one was not such an easy one for me to wrap my brain around at first. I didn't necessarily understand that there was always a difference between *right* and *happy*. I now have a much better understanding of the two words, which has a lot to do with providing to others while doing service work. I could make the choice to be right, but if the cost is my happiness, does it really matter that I was right?

I'll share with you a recent example of this, as I think it will show you how this works. I spend every spare moment

I have with my Mom. She is amazing, and I love being with her, and now with her dementia, it is quite difficult at times (and that is really an understatement!). I have done a lot of reading and research about how to provide the best support and care that I can for her, but when all is said and done, I come back to this: my goal is always to bring her as much happiness as possible. She will often get an idea in her head that is not based on anything factual, yet in her mind, she believes it to be 100 percent true – that is an example of cognitive impairment. So, I have a choice each time I am faced with choosing how I respond to her. I could argue with her and try to convince her that she's wrong and I'm right and what she believes did not really happen, but why would I do that? Everyone benefits when I choose to be *happy* instead of having to be *right*, in spite of such a terrible disease and circumstances. It truly is making the best out of what we have!

Chapter 13

Obstacles in the Way of Living Your Best Life

"The need for change bulldozed a road down the centre of my mind."

Maya Angelou

FORDitude Outcomes

This books content is written in a general way which only scratches the surface as it pertains to the solutions that I discuss in each step. It is through our one on one coaching sessions together; we will get to know each other and build a level of trust and support. This will allow me to delve into your thoughts, feelings, emotions, reactions and goals to understand and most effectively customize the FORDitude daily action program for you.

When Olivia was first introduced to me and showed a real interest in finding out more about my program I hadn't finished writing this manuscript, so I wasn't able to simply hand it to her and say go ahead and good luck. As it turns out, that was a good thing for us both.

During our first meeting, while Olivia was outlining her desired program outcomes, a few things became clear to me:

- She would benefit from having a coach and/or support system during the initial integration of the program in determining how and why setting up a schedule that works is essential for long-term success;

- She benefitted from help in choosing daily and weekly activities until she was more familiar with all of the options;
- Weekly coaching on each step would be useful for her as she implemented them into her life, especially in the critical first few weeks. This helps to ensure success when the brain kicks up a stink because, as we know, it does not like to do new things.

One of my roles as your coach will be to make certain that you are reminded with positive, gentle reinforcement of the rewards of sticking with the changes, and the incredible benefits that will be yours by doing the work and managing your mind! Come check out my website and schedule your free consultation with me today at www.hopeishere.online.

21/90 Crucial Rule

As I stated, especially during the crucial first few weeks of your brain *not* wanting to make these changes, it will take the path of least resistance. It will want to bump the healthy new pathways, putting it back into the old tracks of what you have been doing already and where it feels more comfortable. Your brain doesn't care that it is not healthy and that you are actually trying to replace the behaviours with new and improved ones. Its wiring is left over from eras long gone, and it doesn't know the difference. It just knows that the old ones were easily done, and that is what your brain really wants to do, and it will *really* make it tough for you to keep up the new good work. It takes twenty-one days for your brain to form new tracks for new actions and behaviours. The rule is twenty-one days to form a habit and ninety days to form a new lifestyle. My question to you is this: do you think it would be worthwhile to hire a coach during this process and transition?

Rhetorical Question, Of Course

I have many inspiration framed quotes displayed on shelves and hanging on my walls, and one of my favorites says this, "There are no shortcuts to anyplace worth going!" I could not agree with that statement any more than *absolutely* 100 percent! As Author Stephen Covey writes, "to ensure success, you would do well to begin with the end in mind," and to increase your success rate by implementing FORDitude into your life, no one is better suited than me to take that journey with you. I will help you to navigate the unknown terrain with a recovery roadmap that is tried and tested. I will be your cheerleader and your coach. I will be your biggest encourager, and your biggest advocate. I will help you to do what I have done. I will help you achieve what I have accomplished. I will teach you that you can manage your BPD and love your life in a way you only dreamt possible – because I am doing all of those things today!

As I would love to be coaching you through the FORDitude program, something to consider is that this journey navigating the recovery roadmap is possible with the right mindset – that combination of courage, strength, and positive attitude and I believe and have every confidence that as long as you decide 100% to commit to successfully completing this program – 100% YOU WILL!!!

Definition of Perfectionism

The definition of perfectionism in psychology is as follows: a personality trait characterized by a person's striving for flawlessness and setting high performance standards, accompanied by critical self-evaluations and concerns regarding others' evaluations. It is best conceptualized as a multidimensional characteristic. Perfectionism drives people to attempt to achieve unattainable ideals or unrealistic goals, often leading to depression and low self-esteem.

One of the problems that I have seen repeatedly in people that I have met in recovery over the years is that they all seem to have traits of perfectionism. I used to think that was a good characteristic, until I realized exactly what it means and what it has caused me to do and to feel. It will stop me before I even get started. Do you relate to any or possibly all of the definition above? If so, you may want to revisit this as I did and work towards striving for excellence instead. This may be one of those old beliefs that we can get rid of now??? What do you think?

Life Will Throw You S**t Balls

Life will still throw the occasional s**t ball at you – of course it will – it's still life, but the difference is, you will have tools and know what to do when that happens. When I was still working in HR as a Staffing Consultant, my manager, Bernadette, would tell me how our job as human resource professionals is to deal with all of the s**t. What made us awesome HR professionals, was knowing how to make the s**t "shine", and I guess I still use that philosophy in all aspects of my life as it is still very true regardless of my role.

There will always be stuff to deal with, and the trick is to find a way to make the best of it and to take the s**t and make it work to your advantage so it can shine for you. Why not make it pretty? It's going to be there anyway!

Chapter 14

Manage Your Mind and You Will Transform Your World!

"The reason I started my transformation with the mind first is because you have to see it first and believe it before you start your journey. You have set your mind at a place called W. I. T.. It's 'Whatever It Takes.'
CeCe Peniston

Coaching Goals

Your goals upon completing full complement coaching sessions with Julie Ford are:

- Being able to respond instead of reacting using mindfulness
- Firm establishment of boundaries and setting limits
- Being able to tolerate others' opinions without becoming defensive; if you disagree your reaction is your responsibility
- Developing a healthy skepticism regarding what others say about you, whether it is positive or negative and knowing that either way, it is none of your business; and that your self-esteem is not hinged to it
- Acquire skills to combat your impulsiveness and unhelpful thinking
- Prevent relapses by learning how to move forward to baseline

- Find the crucial individual support you need
- Manage your behaviors so you can give your loved ones the care they need
- Stay functional in your relationships
- Learn how to manage your thinking and emotions no matter what happens

Get Your Butt in the Arena

So, I encourage you to dig as deep as you have to for the courage to get in the arena and look past the reasons that may present themselves to you – remembering **FEAR** is **F**alse **E**vidence **A**ppearing **R**eal. Really ask yourself what you are willing to do to move to the next level in your life. Examine the real reasons you may be too afraid to take a chance and make a change, knowing that it could lead you to the transformation of your whole world changing for the better in ways you couldn't begin to imagine – that is, *until* you get to experience and enjoy them first hand. If you stop and consider a moment, you have to choose whether to be in faith or fear because you can't be in both mindsets at the same time. Make your choice wisely and with the remainder of your life in the forefront of you mind. My personal philosophy has become to make what remains of my life the absolute best of my life, and I invite you to do the same.

In writing my book, it is my greatest hope that through my personal experiences, I was able to convey to you, my reader, that not only is it possible to conquer the devasting effects of BPD, but that you can do it too. Not only can you do it, but you will know that you are worthy of a life you never even dreamt possible. The old tapes of the committee of a**holes, playing on repeat in your head twenty-four hours a day, can and will be replaced by a soundtrack that contains messages of love, acceptance, gratitude, and forgiveness. Your self-doubt will reappear, and you will often forget your worth on your journey. It is important that you continue to have the necessary recovery support in place to ensure that you are able find your way back to your heart and your goodness, quickly, so you do not lose your path as you have done in the past. I have found, in my experience, that the best results have always come when I have been able to work and connect with like-minded people who share understanding, knowledge, experiences, caring, dreams, and goals.

I believe strongly that by adopting the FORDitude program into your life, it will allow you to establish a daily routine, which will ensure you gain the skills to be able to manage the ultimate project: your life. In our coaching sessions, we can design a method to incorporate an effective balance of knowledge, DBT and CBT skills, mindfulness, exercise, positive mindset, connection, and relationship to a purpose greater than yourself. I will show and teach more about how wonderful it is having HOPE (**H**old **O**n **P**ain **E**nds) in your life today, and what it will truly mean for you to *finally* learn how to understand and guide your mind, BPD, and love your life, in a way you never imagined possible.

It all works out in the end and if it doesn't work out, it isn't the end.

Acknowledgments

To my parents, I have so much to give thanks to you for, not the least of which is my life, especially in the early days. It was anything but easy, but I also know that you did the best that you could with what you had to work with. I love you both with my whole heart and thank you for your love when I did everything to push it and you away. I can't even imagine how difficult it was to raise a child like me while dealing with issues of your own. I am so glad to be able to be here for you both every day now, and I am so grateful for your acceptance and support of all that I am and all that I have overcome with all of your help to do so. Without you, I truly don't know where I'd be.

Brianna Elizabeth, you are my reason for getting up every day and my inspiration for all that I do. I can't express how much I love you or what you mean to me, adequately. In my darkest days, I always felt a ray of hope and light, and it was you. You have made each day better, each smile bigger, each joke funnier, and each laugh louder and longer than the one before. There are few people in this world that I truly believe to be witty, smart, and all around awesome just to be in their presence, and you, my love, are one of the rare gems. Thank you for the lessons you don't even realize you teach me daily, the unconditional acceptance you show me, the limitless love you give me, and being an example of the best kind of human being out there. You've made me the proudest mama I could've ever dreamt of being.

To the special folks who have been there, reached out, and shared their medical expertise with me along my path of healing and hope, I can't begin to thank you enough for all you've done and for believing in me when I could not believe in myself.

And to the rest of my chosen tribe of family and friends, in recovery and outside of it, in the rooms, and outside of them, in blood and outside of it, in love and more love because that's all there is – thanks to each and every one of you for your part in my life and in my journey. Without you, there would be a different me. To Angela Lauria and the Team at The Author Incubator – thanks for helping me make a difference! Thank you to Jesse Krieger and the Lifestyle Entrepreneurs Press Publishing team for helping me bring this book to print.

Thank You

I want to take this opportunity to say thank you for reading my book *From Borderline to Baseline*! And, thank you, again, for not giving up on yourself and quitting before you made it all the way through. I have heard it said before, and it is worth repeating here, no one ever said it would be easy, just that it would be worth it. From my own personal recovery experience, I could not agree with that statement more!

And what's more, I believe in you! Why, you might ask? I don't know you – or so you may think – but what I do know is that you haven't fought this hard to give up now. I believe, you were meant to find this book, and with those two things, I would like to offer up a third for you to consider. Once you begin implementing FORDitude in your life, you can keep in touch with me on my website www.hopeishere.online or my Facebook page *From Borderline to Baseline* keep me posted and in the know with how it is working in your life. My questions to you are what do you think is the worst thing that can happen to you? What if things improve for you?

I will be your biggest cheerleader and will be happy to share tips with you along your journey of discovery. I will be able to get to know you and learn more about you along the way. I can suggest helpful videos to watch and informative articles to read. So, one last question – tell me, what have you got to lose? Let's start you loving your life today!

In love and light, Julie

Website: www.hopeishere.online
Facebook: from borderline to baseline
Email: hopeishereonline@outlook.com

About the Author

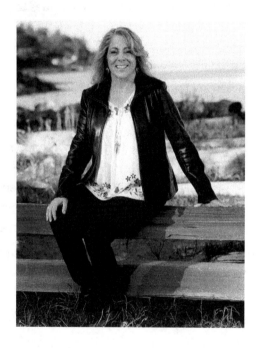

Julie Ann Ford is a transformational author and caregiver who is passionate about helping those affected with BPD. She is the youngest of three daughters born in Halifax, Nova Scotia and, as a military brat, she has lived in many places, including Israel and Egypt.

Julie started on a road of self-discovery that led her to embrace years of sobriety and, more importantly, discover a deep passion for helping others. She finds it very reward-ing and truly loves helping others and has been providing sponsorship to women in recovery from alcoholism for over a decade. Eight years ago, Julie was inspired to create an annual AA weekend campout at Miracle Beach, BC, with the support of a couple friends, that continues to grow in strength and numbers. This legacy is a way of giving back, as her first spiritual awakening and sobriety was found at a similar event.

Julie's greatest joy and accomplishment is her daughter Brianna, her miracle baby. She is the inspiration for Julie sharing her story and creating the FORDitude Daily Action Program, which she developed after recovering from BPD.

Julie sees the road to helping others as a way to shine a light on a lifetime of living with BPD. She is doing everything she can to make the tough road she has lived, and continues to navigate, a lot less difficult for others. She hopes her FORDitude program and personal experiences will give you a roadmap to live a more peaceful, successful life.

CPSIA information can be obtained
at www.ICGtesting.com
Printed in the USA
LVHW050906270121
677550LV00017BB/3078

9 781950 367481